Public Discourse and Health Policies

The questions addressed in the book revolve around the public nature of health as an asset and the rights associated with it, by drawing attention to sociology's role in shedding light on current dynamics and understanding how they may change in the future.

In the field of public health, significant empirical evidence points not only to the outcomes, clinical and otherwise, that extensive information can produce but also to the urgent need to rethink the far from straightforward relationship between having this information and the ability to put it to effective use in tackling the problems it relates to.

The book is intended for a broad audience of university researchers and students, particularly those involved in upper-level sociology and social policy programs. It will also be of interest to healthcare and social work policy-makers and practitioners who wish to gain a more detailed grasp of the dynamics of healthcare in order to approach its processes critically and improve their outcomes.

Nicoletta Bosco is Full Professor of the Sociology of Cultural and Communication Processes at the Department of Cultures, Politics and Society, Università di Torino, Italy.

Routledge Studies in the Sociology of Health and Illness

For more information about this series, please visit: https://www.routledge.com/Routledge-Studies-in-the-Sociology-of-Health-and-Illness/book-series/RSSHI

Public Discourse and Health Policies

The Price of Health in Contemporary Italy

Nicoletta Bosco

Routledge
Taylor & Francis Group
LONDON AND NEW YORK

First published 2022
by Routledge
2 Park Square, Milton Park, Abingdon, Oxon OX14 4RN

and by Routledge
605 Third Avenue, New York, NY 10158

Routledge is an imprint of the Taylor & Francis Group, an informa business

© 2022 Nicoletta Bosco

The right of Nicoletta Bosco to be identified as author of this work has been asserted in accordance with sections 77 and 78 of the Copyright, Designs and Patents Act 1988.

British Library Cataloguing-in-Publication Data
A catalogue record for this book is available from the British Library

Library of Congress Cataloging-in-Publication Data
A catalog record for this book has been requested

ISBN: 978-0-367-42701-6 (hbk)
ISBN: 978-1-032-15709-2 (pbk)
ISBN: 978-0-367-85451-5 (ebk)

DOI: 10.4324/9780367854515

Typeset in Times New Roman
by Apex CoVantage, LLC

Contents

Acknowledgments

Just as the practices involved in public health entail a broad range of different skills, disciplines and approaches, writing a book—even one with a single author—is never just an individual effort. And in the past years, many circumstances and many people have contributed to setting the stage for this volume. The Department of Cultures, Politics and Society of which I am a part has offered—for almost a decade—manifold opportunities for discussing health issues from the whole panorama of perspectives that unfold in this text: those of sociology and anthropology, with their increasingly tight focus on patients' experiences, organizational dimensions and the social representations that contribute to defining them; the political sciences, with their attention to decision processes and deliberative participation, and their call for reflecting on the status of patients' rights; history and the insights it provides for interpreting the present; linguistics with its scrutiny of discourse and the words we use; and social statistics with the tools it provides for using data knowledgeably. My heartfelt thanks also go to my colleagues at the Sociology of Health and Medicine section of the Italian Sociological Association for their commitment to broadening the field's horizons and demonstrating the importance of the sociological outlook in public health. I would thus like to thank all of my colleagues who have added to the debate, as well as those who in the future decide to devote their energies to issues that, with the pandemic, have necessarily taken on new significance for all of us. Another important experience of the past years has been my work with students in the master's degree programs in Sociology and in Anthropology, the postgraduate program in Psychology of Health, and the Ways of Seeing Workshop, whom I would like to thank for their often passionate participation in discussions of communication and health and the many valuable stimuli that they thus afforded me.

Lastly, my affectionate thanks to Andrea Sormano, who was the first to read the entire text, and to Scott Kraemer, the tireless translator thanks to whom the book was undoubtedly improved. Responsibility for the volume's content and limitations, however, is entirely my own.

This book is dedicated to Nicola Negri, mentor, colleague and friend with whom I spent untold hours discussing the original plans for the book and its first chapters. I am sure that—had he been able—he would have willingly continued to discuss the rest as illuminatingly as he has done in all the precious years that I have known him.

Introduction

Information and health in a changing world

In 1849, London was swept by a devastating outbreak of cholera. In ten days, there were over 500 deaths in Broad Street alone. Victorian reformers believed that the outbreak was caused by the city's noxious air and, to investigate its characteristics and risks, a Board of Health committee was appointed to collect all possible information: from the variations in atmospheric pressure and the winds to household ventilation conditions. No credit was given to an equally sizable collection of empirical evidence amassed at the time by the physician John Snow, who argued—rightly—that cholera was spread by contaminated water (Farr, 1852). Despite this evidence to the contrary, the measures that were taken embraced the common-sense explanation that was widespread in the period, demonstrating that information *per se* does not necessarily lead to a better awareness of the action that should be taken, but can, under certain circumstances, reinforce existing ways of framing a problem. Indeed, when we find ourselves facing alternative explanations for an unknown phenomenon, what information we should trust is not always clear even to the experts, especially when we are aware of the risks that the wrong decision would bring.

Although many years have passed since then—and it is now widely recognized that we must often cook up our decisions from a hodgepodge of disparate ingredients rather than any objective knowledge of proven facts—the growing production of information and the increasing ease of access to it have tended to reinstate an unreflecting model of the relationship between knowledge and decision-making.

It is undoubtedly reassuring to think of how many changes in our knowledge of physical and physiological matters have taken place in all the years that insulate us from what life was like in mid-nineteenth-century London. And these changes are a key part of the story we are about to tell. At least in the Western world, a growing proportion of the population has been fortunate enough to live unburdened with worries about what it means to be ill or to risk illness, often for much of their lives. Many—though by no means all—of the factors that contributed to this happy state will figure in the following pages: better diagnostic capabilities, new drugs and treatment, longer life expectancy and the progressive institutionalization of Europe's healthcare systems, especially in the so-called "Glorious Thirty", the

DOI: 10.4324/9780367854515-1

years between the end of the Second World War and the mid-1970s. But over time, blind faith in steady progress and the results it hoped to bring proved misplaced. Closer to our own days, troubling evidence has mounted about new, worldwide problems exacerbated by the 2007 financial crisis. Drastically worsening environmental conditions, the concentration of wealth in fewer and fewer hands, the growing masses of the poor, soaring joblessness, a shrinking social safety net, and widening health inequalities in access to drugs and treatment for acute and chronic illnesses amount to "a savage sorting", bringing complex modes of expulsion that have denied rights and sustainable living conditions for unprecedented swaths of the population, even in the richest countries (Sassen, 2014). Around the world, the picture on the eve of the pandemic in early 2020 was one of widespread fragility and risk, with millions of people facing the prospects of worse to come. Despite the undeniable and, in many ways, astonishing advances made by science, it must be admitted that things have not gone as expected, and that the global situation is evolving in a direction that calls for greater attention to the many questions surrounding the possibilities for using our knowledge to support public health.

1 An emergency foretold

This book, which addresses the issues associated with health and the communication processes involved in health decisions and the public debate, took shape against a backdrop which, in some ways, seems unique, though in reality it raises age-old questions and touches on problems that are anything but new. The first question regards predictability. Why, despite the increase in knowledge about the causal mechanisms behind the insurgence and spread of diseases and infections, were we not better able to see what was coming?

The World Health Organization itself has pointed out how ambivalent the current situation is: "The COVID-19 pandemic is in many respects unprecedented, but in no respect was it unforeseen" (WHO, 2021, p. VI). Over the years, many signs that a pandemic might be in the offing drew attention to the need for a global warning, alert and emergency response system to fend off what could very well be a catastrophe. In 2005, WHO researchers issued the following statement:

> During 2004, concern about the threat of a pandemic set in motion a number of activities, coordinated by WHO, that are leaving the world better prepared for the next pandemic, whenever it occurs and whichever virus causes it. Nonetheless, our highly mobile and interconnected world remains extremely vulnerable. No one can say whether the present situation will turn out to be another narrow escape or the prelude to the first pandemic of the 21st century. Should the latter event occur, we must not be caught unprepared.
>
> (WHO, 2005, p. 3)

In the following years, between 2014 and 2016, events such as the Ebola hemorrhagic fever outbreak in West Africa once again riveted experts' attention, and in

September 2019 the Global Preparedness Monitoring Board—made up of specialists from the World Bank and the WHO—launched another alarm:

> Disease thrives in disorder and has taken advantage—outbreaks have been on the rise for the past several decades and the spectre of a global health emergency looms large. If it is true to say "what's past is prologue", then there is a very real threat of a rapidly moving, highly lethal pandemic of a respiratory pathogen killing 50 to 80 million people and wiping out nearly 5% of the world's economy.
>
> (GPMB, September 2019, p. 6)

It should be pointed out that calls to gird for emergencies, and the growing body of documented evidence about them, do not automatically produce any real idea of what "preparedness" means and what concrete action should be taken to achieve it (Mangesho et al., 2021). That all the signals indicated that a pandemic was certain to come, and the only unknowns were when and where, brings us to a factor that was to prove central in the current state of affairs, viz., the difficulty in determining what the right policy choices may be in a zero-sum situation where resources are clearly inadequate even to cope with business as usual:

> Preparedness for a pandemic presents a dilemma: what priority should be given to an unpredictable but potentially catastrophic event, when many existing and urgent health needs remain unmet?
>
> (WHO, 2005, p. 3)

Belying expectations about the collective capacity to keep health risks in check, and despite years of credible predictions, the epidemic that spread around the globe at the beginning of 2020 (or even earlier, as some believe) demonstrated that the response to the priority dilemma posed by the WHO failed to come up with preparedness plans for an emergency that was widely held to be only a question of time (Zichitella, 2020).

2 An unprecedented emergency

Saying that the pandemic was predictable is not the same as denying that it is exceptional. This brings us close to the crux of what we will be dealing with in the book, and in particular to the convoluted relationship between knowing, not knowing and deciding. Compared to past pandemics, Covid-19 has certain specific features that made responding to the emergency even more complicated, though we are also better able to predict and treat illness. A mixture of biological and epidemiological factors has contributed to making the current pandemic exceptional—the virus' transmissibility and lethality, for instance—while the context in which it spread has also played a part. Regarding the first set of aspects, the virus is more readily transmitted (and this seems even truer of its recent variants) and less lethal than other viruses such as Ebola, which kill their hosts more quickly and thus have less time to infect others.

The second set of factors that make the current pandemic exceptional has to do with the social aspects that helped it spread. It almost goes without saying that globalization and the increasing ease with which goods and people circulate throughout the planet have made the virus' movements harder to track and contain. Less obvious—and harder to reconstruct—is the role of politics in the virus' spread. Politics, however, establish priorities and mediate between the many actors and interests on the national and international scene in order to ensure that levels of procurement match the size of the problems that arise. This makes it all the more urgent to consider the effects of a composite set of factors, social as well as biomedical, that are central to public health (Horton, 2020). Suddenly, the sheer scope of the Covid-19 pandemic has radically changed allocation decisions: "never before have so many resources been directed to manage the spread and impact of a single medical condition in such a short period of time" (Manderson & Wahlberg, 2020, p. 434). The upshot is that the population affected by other conditions is more fragile than before, both because those living with chronic diseases are more vulnerable to the virus, and because many forms of treatment have been postponed or cut back as hospitals and wards have shut down non-Covid operations to concentrate on the pandemic. Similarly, these vulnerable patients have canceled outpatient visits or delayed seeking emergency treatment for fear of contracting the virus. The combined effect is to put patients in a considerable quandary:

> During COVID-19 lockdowns, both caregivers and those with serious non-communicable diseases must adjudicate conflicting messages and perform their own triage: to remain in isolation and allow time to determine outcome (hoping either that certain symptoms will subside and prove unimportant, or that restrictions on everyday social interactions will be lifted); or seek help as symptoms may become crises demanding action despite risk. Ironically, they are "at risk" of their known conditions while in self-isolation to protect themselves from the virus they are "at risk" of dying from.
>
> (Manderson & Wahlberg, 2020, p. 432)

In addition to the unprecedented problems in how to allocate available resources and patient's new but more-than-legitimate concerns, other ways in which the pandemic has put us on unfamiliar ground have depended on the nature, relationships and balance of power between national and international organizations. These dynamics and their often unpredictable outcomes have involved equally complex phenomena, such as the changes in the World Health Organization as the resources provided by its member states have been increasingly outweighed by donations from the great private charitable foundations (Dentico & Missoni, 2021). As Dentico, who heads the Society for International Development (SID) Global Health Program, points out, the International Health Regulations formulated after the

2005 SARS emergency laid down specific requirements for cooperation between countries during health crises, but almost nothing has been done despite urging on the part of the WHO Director-General and repeated calls for solidarity: "governments either hide the numbers or do not cooperate with each other, and are—still now, unfortunately—in denial. For the virus, this is the perfect storm" (interview with N. Dentico in Zichitella, 2020). Laggard cooperation is nowhere more apparent than in the case of vaccine distribution: as of the end of February 2021, over 50% of all vaccine doses had been purchased by high-income countries that account for only 16% of the world's population (Yamey, 2021).

The pandemic has brought yet another set of circumstances to light. The difficulty in deciding on priorities—and the not necessarily unquestioned authority wielded by those who should make these decisions—makes it even harder to determine the best ways of communicating these choices to ensure that they are acceptable to the public.

In the following pages, we will be looking at the role of communication processes in dealing with health questions of central importance to the community and the many ambivalent links between decision-making and available information. This is another area where we should have been on more familiar ground when the pandemic struck. Writing on the last century's Spanish flu, the historian John Barry acknowledged: "In the next influenza pandemic, be it now or in the future, be the virus mild or virulent, the single most important weapon against the disease will be a vaccine. The second most important will be communication" (Barry, 2009; Villa, 2014).

Making sense of something as extraordinary as the Covid pandemic and finding a way to navigate through it calls for a thorough rethinking of our usual ideas about health and illness under less extreme conditions. And this brings us to two further points: the first is that there is an urgent need to find answers that can help us deal with health issues; the second concerns the opportunities arising from a change of perspective that has suddenly put healthcare in the spotlight after many decades (since the 1980s at the very least) of disregard and dwindling resources had threatened its nature as a public good.

3 Reconceptualizing health: syndemics and remission society

Our remarks so far have suggested that public health should be observed in terms of its multiple, interconnecting levels, from a broad perspective that also encompasses the social, economic, political and interpersonal aspects that together contribute to defining health, the choices made to preserve public health, the representations that take shape and the communication processes that—intentionally or otherwise—bring them before the public eye.

To take aim at the unexplored implications of what is now going on, and to take a closer look at the form that greater attention to communication about health and its public nature could take (Conrad & Barker, 2010), we will draw on two concepts: that of syndemic conditions (Singer & Clair, 2003) and the need for a wider recognition of the inevitable fragility of human existence.

The term syndemic was introduced by the medical anthropologist Merrill Singer in the 1990s in reference to the need for a clinical approach that takes into account the adverse synergistic interactions of co-present diseases—disease–disease interaction—sustained by the social context in which they occur (social condition interaction):

> this concept moves beyond common medical conceptualisations of comorbidity and multimorbidity—when diseases simply occur in tandem—because it both concerns the consequences of disease interaction and the social, environmental, or economic factors that cluster with the diseases and shape their interaction.
>
> (Singer et al., 2017, pp. 941–942)

Being able to identify these interactions is an important prerequisite for determining the prognosis of these diseases and treating them effectively as well as for formulating broad-based health policies:

> The syndemics orientation has the potential to affect health policy by drawing attention to how social, economic, and environmental factors affect the health of human beings, provided that these factors are not separated in analysis from disease emergence or comorbidity. Instead, the clustering of diseases and the vulnerability of populations to disease must be recognised to incorporate inherent social and environmental risk factors.
>
> (Singer et al., 2017, p. 946)

The syndemics approach—and the relational perspective underlying it—assumes that in order to deal with a given condition caused, for example, by a pandemic infection, it is not enough to treat the patients who contract the disease. It is also necessary to employ multicausal, multifactorial models:

> In medicine, for example, an ageing population requires management of individuals not just with multiple comorbid diseases but also with pronounced interacting diseases and compromising social conditions, such as impoverishment or social isolation. Given that social conditions can contribute to the formation, clustering, and progression of disease, a biosocial concept like syndemics offers a holistic approach to addressing synergistic disease and context interactions. Syndemic theory seeks to draw attention to and to provide a framework for the analysis of these kinds of biosocial connections, including their causes and consequences for human life and wellbeing, and for responding with appropriate intervention.
>
> (Singer et al., 2017, p. 942)

The second concept underpinning the thrust of this book is that of the remission society. Frank uses this expression for the many people who, at some point in their lives, have had a close encounter with illness, or even a near-death experience and, though their symptoms are in remission, are nevertheless both more exposed but also more aware of their frailty:

> Members of the remission society include those who have had almost any cancer, those living in cardiac recovery programs, diabetics, those whose allergies and environmental sensitivities require dietary and other self-monitoring, those with protheses and mechanical body regulators, the chronically ill, the disabled, those "recovering" from abuses and addictions, and for all these people, the families that share the worries and daily triumph of staying well.
>
> (Frank, 2013, p. 8)

Belonging to this group means being separated from the rest of society by a deep divide. At the same time, however, its members must construct a newly defined self and activate their so-called negative capabilities (Lanzara, 1993), the skills needed to live with fear and uncertainty and, for those who have been ill, entail "a constant balancing between health and illness, and being either in and out of control" (Ellingsen et al., 2021, p. 35).

What do all of us, today, have in common with this society of sufferers? Frank's description of how illness pulls the carpet out from underneath everyday existence chimes in many ways with how we have lived as a result of the pandemic, whose effects have extended the individual experiences of those coping with chronic illness to all of our communities, unwilling enrollees in the remission society. The pandemic has made all of us familiar with the fears, qualms and uncertainties of those who find themselves catapulted into an unknown universe, where the maps we live by no longer apply. Many narratives of the pandemic—as told by Covid patients, their families, their nurses and doctors—describe the bewilderment felt when so many things we were used to, socialized to—being close, sharing, hugs, taking care of a sick family member—suddenly became risky or wrong (Giordano, 2020). Fear is our fellow-traveler, ever-present, making it hard even to image a return to some nominal normality whose contours are still foggy. But there is also an inkling of optimism, a bet on a better future, in this extension of the notion of the remission society to our pandemic experience: "Illness remains a nightmare in many ways, but it also becomes a possibility, especially for a more intimate connection with others" (Frank, 2013, p. XV). Replacing the word illness with pandemic gives us a rough idea of the conditions we would willingly have forgone that were created in healthcare, but which so forcefully brought home the need to recenter attention on rights, on what frailty is and how to support it, on the importance of health as a public good and on appropriate ways to safeguard and promote it. Like chronic illness' daily grind, the pandemic and the uncertainty it brought are an incentive to rethink health and its functions and structures to gain a clearer grasp of its determinants and where it ranks among other spheres of public life:

> One cannot have an epidemic without an organising system that categorises—sometimes explicitly and often implicitly—what counts as disease and where it belongs: whether in certain countries, bodies, ages, or even historical periods. Throwing up bewildering challenges to widespread and triumphalist views of modern-day exceptionalism, epidemics represent crises of social order, where pathogens are displaced from where they "belong" and states of health are disordered from where they "should be." They risk upending an often fragile collective acceptance of the dominant classification system, and in doing so they generate uncertainty, fear, and conflict. Attempts to rectify the crisis invariably expose fault-lines within a society—frequently amplifying differences in categories such as able-bodiedness, age, class, ethnicity, gender, race, and sexuality—and offer insights into its explicit and implicit value systems.
>
> (Charter & McKay, 2020, p. 227)

Drawing on the concept of the remission society does not mean assuming that there is a widespread awareness of what is going on and the impact it will have on our lives nor does it mean believing that our suffering will be our redemption. Fear, or the awareness of danger, will often get us nowhere. It thus cannot be taken for granted that our pandemic experiences will trigger any ability to redefine our lives and try, as Frank urges the members of the remission society to do, to find: "*how to live a good life while being ill*" (2013, p. 156, emphasis in original). Extending the concept of the remission society to the conditions brought by the pandemic, we can rephrase this as "how to live the best possible life given the circumstances". Understanding if and how this is possible calls for an analytical approach that combines the biomedical outlook with what Kleinman, Eisenberg and Good have called the cultural construction of clinical reality (1978). This approach has been widely evoked over the years, but it is always difficult to implement since it involves keeping track of the transactions between the actors' many different explanatory models, therapeutic values, expectations and goals: "Clinical realities are thus culturally constructed and vary cross-culturally and across the domains of health care in the same society" (Kleinman et al., 1978, p. 144).

But there are multiple signs that many things are not going as might be hoped, and that the current situation demonstrates that we cannot assume that our knowledge will ever segue smoothly into the choices we make. At the macro level, we have mentioned the scant coordination between countries and the resistance to implementing health emergency plans on a global scale. As for the reactions on the part of the public, many have been dysfunctional: the increase in domestic violence during lockdowns (de Borba Telles et al., 2020; Piquero et al., 2021), attacks on vaccination centers, anti-lockdown protests (Haddad, 2021) and higher levels of depression and mental health problems (Daly et al., 2020; Fegert et al., 2020) all bring troubling questions about the collective ability to weather the crisis and to accept and come to grips with the remission society's implications. In addition to acting on their fears, the public has also shown other signs of denial and coping strategies. The increase in the numbers of people in many countries seeking cosmetic surgery or requesting teleconsultations with plastic surgeons during the pandemic (Padley & Di Pace, 2021) is an example of how priorities and preferences can be juggled in unexpected ways, and how a distraction can seem to be an attractive escape route, allowing us to shirk the urgent questions we should be facing.

Were we living in a rational world, we would have expected that the pandemic's predictability would have enabled us to get ready for it. It would also have been legitimate to expect that tackling the pandemic would not have diverted the healthcare institutions' attention away from the inescapable baseline of illness, or that we, as members of the public, would have been able to arrive at a more prudent and informed assessment of how to conduct ourselves. But however reasonable such a linear conception of the relationship between information, knowledge and choices would have been, this is not what came to pass:

> Given these insights from decades of anthropological research, it is conspicuous that discussions of the management of pandemics—not only COVID-19 but also Zika, Ebola, and H1N1 before it—take little account of preexisting conditions other than as an indicator of vulnerability of serious infection and death.
>
> (Manderson & Wahlberg, 2020, p. 431)

As we look for an answer to why this should have been, the book will discuss the discourses and representations surrounding the health system, breaking them down into their component parts and reconstructing their determinants, not from the stories of people who have experienced illness but from the narratives that take shape around them, the actors who put these narratives into circulation and the mechanisms that they generate. In chronicling these aspects of the health systems, our aim is to understand where we are today, and where we could and should go to get back on track. We will thus be exploring the way contexts shape public discourses about health, from what is named and visible, to what is never openly mentioned but reveals its presence in the practices that come to be adopted.

Rethinking old certainties and priorities about health, and finding ways to discuss and defend the choices that could be made are both possible and necessary but not—as we will see—free from risks and ambiguities. Inevitably, the urgency of refocusing on the conditions necessary for global health creates a sense of uncertainty and anxiety. And as each of us, individually, knows from experience, uncertainty, urgency and anxiety are not conducive to making good decisions about complex matters.

In a world where many familiar landmarks have crumbled, we need some other way of getting our bearings: new maps and new compasses. As we explore the world of health here, however, we will not follow a single lodestar, but will venture into many of the byways that beckon to us on our way, at the risk of seeming at times to lose sight of the broader horizon. It will be a voyage of discovery, continually unearthing ideas and conceptions of health, some new, some familiar, some forgotten or lost by the wayside.

But voyages are part of our discipline. The social sciences themselves not infrequently find themselves traversing unknown or ill-charted territory, a fact that demonstrates—for once with no need for further explanation or justification—the weight and the inevitable interconnections between theory and practice, and the rightful role of both in helping us understand uncertainty and the plural and situated ways in which human beings try to deal with it.

As we will see, tracking the problems we face in re-centering attention on health will mean penetrating deep into territories that are often passed over, unnoticed.

4 What we'll be talking about in the book

In the field of public health, significant empirical evidence points not only to the outcomes, clinical and otherwise, that extensive information can produce but also to the urgent need to rethink the far from straightforward relationship between having information and being able or willing to put it to effective use in tackling the problems it relates to.

What are the mechanisms that can help us understand the yawning gap separating the expectations of continual improvement in the systems that deal with our health from the suboptimal situations we see today? How is healthcare systems' performance evaluated, and what makes it so difficult to reach a consensus on what should be done to safeguard aspects that are so central to our wellbeing? What do we talk about and what do we take for granted in discussions of health and the choices to be made, and what remains unsaid? How are the priorities for allocating resources set, and how are they communicated?

To answer the many questions surrounding information and decisions in healthcare, the book will begin by discussing why the Italian National Health Service's scores in the international rankings do not shed light on its operation or the changes affecting it. Average performance figures, in fact, conceal major disparities—regional and otherwise—that call for a detailed analysis, distinguishing between effects springing from the fact that many different interests are involved, and the unintended effects that are now coming to the fore, unforeseen by the stakeholders. Our discussion of the Italian situation will introduce the criteria used to define the quality of healthcare systems and the question of whether there can indeed be a straightforward link between having information and putting it to good use in formulating policies. The fact that Italy's regional healthcare systems vary widely from region to region, and the regions themselves are very different in terms of wealth distribution and GDP, casts a certain amount of doubt on how much reliance can be put on scores based on national averages. And yet, rankings seem to have a strange ability to command credence. If placing near the top in a healthcare system performance report is a guarantee of quality, how is it that some countries have very high scores in some ranking systems and very low ones in others? For a closer look at how the indicators we choose affect what we are describing and the effects that are produced, Chapter 2 scrutinizes the theoretical aspects of the rocky road that links decision-making, public policy and policy justification in governance processes. Collective narratives are at the center of political life, given that problems—and the ways of tacking them—are not accepted on the basis of intrinsic and universally acknowledged values. Rather, human action is understood on the basis of images, representations and systems of expectations that can be considered appropriate or less so, and thus must strive to convince. Here, the central factors include the ambiguous role played by the information underpinning decisions, and the reasons that may result in incomplete information (e.g., incorrect use of data, either intentional or unintentional, underestimating unexpected events, gaming strategies or the difficulty of striking a balance between short- and long-term consequences). These issues are relevant well beyond Italy's borders, as witnessed by the extensive international literature on decision-making processes, public policy choices and the justifications offered for them. These aspects are especially important in spheres such as healthcare that should be subject to specific safeguards because of the consequences they can have on public life. Information is central, and whether it is accepted hinges, to a large extent, on how it is constructed and circulated. While up-to-date and accurate information is crucial, it is equally crucial that its characteristics, its sources, who provide it and how it is used are clear. Nevertheless, ensuring that the criteria behind choices are transparent is not always smooth sailing, and not all choices can be discussed publicly without running into problems.

The third chapter addresses the "tragic choices" that must be made in healthcare, for example, how to distribute resources when there are not enough to go around. These are not problems that arise only in emergencies like the pandemic. More often than one might think, in fact, resources are inadequate even in the best of times, and it is thus necessary to determine what allocation criteria will be used and find ways of making them as broadly acceptable as possible. But this is often fraught with knotty questions, ethical and otherwise. How do we decide what a life is worth? Who sets the price? And what about the lives whose value we have chosen not to acknowledge? Letting it be known that we will leave someone behind is not easy: no one wants to be denied a resource their survival could depend on. To demonstrate how complex these decisions are and how difficult it is to communicate their outcomes, the chapter will outline the main selection criteria, the ideas underlying them and the many different principles at their root. In doing so, it will discuss the dilemmas the processes in question pose, the difficulties of bringing them into the public debate and the concrete attempts that have been made in various parts of the world—through the use of deliberative strategies, for example—to pass from theory to practice. The chapter concludes with a brief overview of the Italian media's coverage of health and healthcare systems in the first stage of the pandemic. As we will see, the tragic choices were passed over almost in silence, just as there was virtually no discussion of public health choices and what the alternatives might have been. Though communication inevitably plays a central part in legitimizing public choices, there was a tendency to ignore the most controversial or painful aspects of the pandemic, essentially preventing media discourses from performing a service in extending the debate on the problems to be tackled. Explicitly or not, the discourses and practices surrounding healthcare and its organization reveal conceptions of health and how it should be pursued that deserve greater attention. Capping our exploration of the disconnects between choices and their underlying assumptions, the fourth chapter reviews the main definitions of health that have been formulated over the years and the processes of naturalization that have enabled some ideas to gain sway over others. The relationship between experts and the public, the dominant conceptions of science that claim to be self-evident are, on closer inspection, the product of processes that are rather more roundabout than might be thought. To investigate these processes, we propose a model of the intersections between the conceptions of science (along a line running through the two poles of science and anti-scientism) and the more or less authoritative role of those who lay down the coordinates of what science is and is not. Though simplified, this model encompasses very different spheres, in which science may be rigid and dogmatic, or open to dialog with all components of society. In these different spheres, what we know, as well as what we do not know or do not want to know, influences the forms communication can take and the effects it can have in a variety of ways. In conclusion, we will touch on a number of open questions and on the need for greater attention to problem-setting in healthcare before proceeding posthaste to problem-solving. This is an area where the social sciences can make a vital contribution in reconstructing the processes whereby meanings and representations are constructed, returning to the idea of possible change and the values and perspectives that can help us pursue it.

References

Barry, J. (2009). Pandemics: Avoiding the Mistakes of 1918. *Nature, 459,* 324–325. https://doi.org/10.1038/459324a.

Charters, E., & McKay, R. A. (2020). The History of Science and Medicine in the Context of COVID-19. *Centaurus, 62,* 223–233. https://doi.org/10.1111/1600-0498.12311.

Conrad, P., & Barker, K. K. (2010). The Social Construction of Illness: Key Insights and Policy Implications. *Journal of Health and Social Behavior, 51*(1_suppl), S67–S79. https://doi.org/10.1177/0022146510383495.

Daly, M., Sutin, A. R., & Robinson, E. (2020). Longitudinal Changes in Mental Health and the COVID-19 Pandemic: Evidence from the UK Household Longitudinal Study. *Psychological Medicine,* 1–10. https://doi.org/10.1017/S0033291720004432.

de Borba, Telles, L. E., Valença, A. M., Barros, A. J. S., & da Silva, A. G. (2020). Domestic Violence in the COVID-19 Pandemic: A Forensic Psychiatric Perspective. *Brazilian Journal of Psychiatry,* Epub 1 June 2020. https://doi.org/10.1590/1516-4446-2020-1060.

Dentico, N., & Missoni, E. (2021). *Geopolitica della salute. Covid-19, OMS e la sfida pandemica.* Soveria Mannelli: Rubbettino Editore.

Ellingsen, S., Moi, A. L., Gjengedal, E., Flinterud, S. I., Natvik, E., Råheim, M., . . . Sekse, R. J. T. (2021). "Finding Oneself After Critical Illness": Voices from the Remission Society. *Medicine, Health, Care and Philosophy*, *24*, 35–44. https://doi.org/10.1007/s11019-020-09979-8.

Farr, W. (1852). *Report on the Mortality of Cholera in England 1848–1849*. London: Great Britain General Register Office.

Fegert, J. M., Vitiello, B., Plener, P. L., & Clemens, V. (2020). Challenges and Burden of the Coronavirus 2019 (COVID-19) Pandemic for Child and Adolescent Mental Health: A Narrative Review to Highlight Clinical and Research Needs in the Acute Phase and the Long Return to Normality. *Child and Adolescent Psychiatry and Mental Health*, *14*, 20. https://doi.org/10.1186/S13034-020-00329-3.

Frank, A. F. (2013). *The Wounded Storyteller. Body, Illness, and Ethics*, Second Edition. Chicago and London: The University of Chicago Press.

Giordano, P. (2020). *Nel contagio*. Torino: Giulio Einaudi Editore.

GPMB. (2019). *A World at Risk: Annual Report on Global Preparedness for Health Emergencies*. https://apps.who.int/gpmb/assets/annual_report/GPMB_annualreport_2019.pdf

Haddad, M. (2021). *Mapping Coronavirus Anti-Lockdown Protests Around the World*, February. www.aljazeera.com/news/2021/2/2/mapping-coronavirus-anti-lockdown-protests-around-the-world.

Horton, R. (2020). Offline: COVID-19 Is Not a Pandemic. *The Lancet*, *396*(10255), 874. https://doi.org/10.1016/S0140-6736(20)32000-6.

Kleinman, A., Eisenberg, L., & Good, B. (1978). Culture, Illness, and Care: Clinical Lessons from Anthropologic and Cross-Cultural Research. *Annals of Internal Medicine*, *88*(2), 251–258. https://doi.org/10.7326/0003-4819-88-2-251.

Lanzara, G. F. (1993). *Capacità negativa. Competenza progettuale e modelli di intervento nelle organizzazioni*. Bologna: il Mulino.

Manderson, L., & Wahlberg, A. (2020). Chronic Living in a Communicable World. *Medical Anthropology*, *39*(5), 428–439. https://doi.org/10.1080/01459740.2020.1761352.

Mangesho, P. E., Caudell, M. A., Mwakapeje, E. R., Ole-Neselle, M., Kimani, T., Dorado-García, A., Kabali, E., & Fasina, F. O. (2021). Knowing Is Not Enough: A Mixed-Methods Study of Antimicrobial Resistance Knowledge, Attitudes, and Practises Among Maasai Pastoralists. *Frontiers in Veterinary Science*, *8*, 645851. https://doi.org/10.3389/fvets.2021.645851.

Padley, R. H., & Di Pace, B. (2021). Touch-ups, Rejuvenation, Re-dos and Revisions: Remote Communication and Cosmetic Surgery on the Rise. *Aesthetic Plastic Surgery*. https://doi.org/10.1007/s00266-021-02235-1.

Piquero, A., Jennings, W. G., Jeminson, E., Kaukinen, C., & Knaul, F. M. (2021). *Domestic Violence During COVID-19 Evidence from a Systematic Review and Meta-Analysis*. Washington, DC: Council on Criminal Justice, March. https://cdn.ymaws.com/counciloncj.org/resource/resmgr/covid_commission/Domestic_Violence_During_COV.pdf.

Sassen, S. (2014). *Expulsions: Brutality and Complexity in the Global Economy*. Cambridge: Harvard University Press.

Singer, M., Bulled, N., Ostrach, B., & Mendenhall, E. (2017). Syndemics and the Biosocial Conception of Health. *Lancet (London, England)*, *389*(10072), 941–950. https://doi.org/10.1016/S0140-6736(17)30003-X.

Singer, M., & Clair, S. (2003). Syndemics and Public Health: Reconceptualizing Disease in Bio-Social Context. *Medical Anthropology Quarterly*, *17*(4), 423–441. https://doi.org/10.1525/maq.2003.17.4.423.

Villa, R. (2014). La comunicazione vale come un vaccino. *Pagina⁹⁹we*, 27 September.

WHO. (2005). *Avian Influenza: Assessing the Pandemic Threat*. https://apps.who.int/iris/bitstream/handle/10665/68985/WHO_CDS_2005.29.pdf;jsessionid.

WHO. (2021). *COVID-19 Strategic Preparedness and Response Plan*. www.who.int/publications/i/item/WHO-WHE-2021.02.

Yamey, G. (2021). Rich Countries Should Tithe Their Vaccines. Game Theory Suggests That Donating Doses Can Help Nations of All Income Levels. *Nature*, 24 February. www.nature.com/articles/d41586-021-00470-9.

Zichitella, R. (2020). É la pandemia più annunciata della storia. *Famiglia Cristiana*. www.famigliacristiana.it/articolo/e-la-pandemia-piu-annunciata-della-storia.aspx.

Chapter 1

International health service rankings

Reflections from an Italian perspective

Whether it's a question of choosing a university, buying a big-ticket item like a car or picking a restaurant, being able to range all of our options along some kind of continuum has an undoubted allure. We're attracted by the idea that the choices we make are based on a knowledge—as complete and rational as possible—of the opportunities available to us and the advantages or disadvantages they bring. Knowing all about the alternatives (or at least thinking we do) strikes us as being a prerequisite for making well-thought-out decisions and holding the uncertainty that any decision inevitably entails in check. And this is all the more important when choices must be made in areas—like individual and collective health—that are central in our own lives and the contexts we live in. Knowing that the physician who is treating us has a good professional reputation, or that the hospital he or she works in and the health service that lays out the coordinates is well-regarded gives us a sense of reassurance that can contribute at least a bit to soothing the anxieties and foreboding that always come with having the symptoms of an illness and not yet knowing whether it's something we should worry about and, if so, how much.

Having access to information about healthcare services' performance is thus a particularly attractive prospect, not just for the individual. On a different scale, being able to compare other countries' systems or services and facilities that compete in the same context can serve, for example, in reallocating public resources and investments, as well as to justify a particular organizational setup or call it into question.

As we will see in the following pages, our need for reassurance or our idea of a world where decisions seem to be carefully weighed on the basis of full, objective and impartial information hardly matches the world we actually live in. For a better knowledge of how systems as complex as those involved in healthcare operate and to understand the relationship between recognizing problems and their scope on the one hand, and their representations and the policies fielded in order to deal with them on the other, it is useful to analyze a concrete case or, in other words, take a case study approach. Here, our case—the Italian situation—provides an excellent vantage point for scrutinizing the mechanisms that can arise: it enables us to observe the different perspectives taken by the actors involved and reflect on

DOI: 10.4324/9780367854515-2

how the meaning of complex constructs such as the quality and organization of healthcare can vary according to the differing goals and viewpoints of those who participate in it. Looking at Italy's position in the international rankings thus opens up a broader perspective that enables us, by exploring differences and similarities, to pinpoint the arguments behind public choices and reflect on the many reasons for the plurality of interests and the views that accompany them. Above all, however, it helps us address what it is that different social settings (and the actors in them) consider valuable, what they believe should be collectively acknowledged as important, and what, conversely, goes unnoticed (McKee & Stuckler, 2011). Depending on the objectives, interests and value orientations of those who are in a position to make decisions about the system's organization and any changes to be made, the indicators chosen to describe how the system operates reflect (and to some extent naturalize) what is regarded as important and must thus be monitored and, inasmuch as is possible, publicly justified. In the case of health (and, obviously, also in other publicly important sectors like the labor market, education or the environment), what constitutes a problem, and what relationship should be established between the discourses about problems and how they are translated into policies is particularly crucial: if an area is considered valuable, then it is necessary that the rationale underlying the choices be clearly understood, along with the actors whom we feel can legitimately express themselves and take action, and the objectives and priorities that are to be pursued. Otherwise, the spotlights either do not go on or are switched off, information either does not circulate or is reduced to a trickle, and issues struggle to come to the fore and consequently are not addressed. In the following pages, we will have a look at how the health field is faring in this connection.

1 A case study: Italy's standing in the international health service rankings

To mark the Italian National Health Service's 40th anniversary in 2018, researchers at GIMBE, the Italian Group for Evidence-Based Medicine (Cartabellotta et al., 2018), a nonprofit group that has monitored the service for years, published a report on how it is viewed in the major international rankings. A number of significant points emerge from the report: while the scores assigned to the Italian National Health Service's performance vary widely, some ranking systems arrive at similar scores even though they consider different aspects. Given that—as we will see—the score or the standing obtained in a ranking is by no means without consequences, looking at each ranking system's characteristics will enable us to begin to get a grasp of the far from predictable nature of the representations of topics of such importance to the collectivity as the health system's organization and outcomes. We will start from two ratings for the situation in 2014. The report by the multinational Bloomberg (2014) puts Italy in first place among European health services, and third among the 51 countries included in the survey. Also, on the basis of 2014 data, the ranking in the Report on Public Finances issued by the

European Commission's Directorate-General for Economic and Financial Affairs (2016) considers indicators of efficiency[1] and effectiveness[2] in the 28 EU member states, and here again Italy is one of the highest-scoring countries together with France, Spain, Ireland, Cyprus and Malta. In this second ranking, the range of efficiency indicators includes the ten-year average of per capita total current expenditure, while the effectiveness indicators include measures such as the amenable mortality rate, the infant mortality rate, life expectancy at birth and life expectancy at 65.

Although the two rankings refer to the same year and agree in assigning a good score to Italy, the snapshot of the country that they give us is taken from angles that overlap only in part. The Bloomberg report sets out to measure the efficiency of each country's health system through three criteria: life expectancy (which accounts for 60% of the ranking); relative cost of healthcare as a percentage of per capita GDP (30%) and absolute per capita cost of healthcare (10%). For each criterion, 80% of the score is derived from the most recent year's performance and 20% on the basis of changes over the previous year. It should be pointed out that neither the choice of criteria nor the weights assigned to each can be regarded as necessary or inevitable. It is obvious, for instance, that life expectancies are likely to (also) depend on conditions that have nothing to do with how well the health service operates, but reflect other factors. American studies conducted in the last century estimated that the services delivered by the healthcare system contribute to increasing life expectancy by only 10%, as against 30% for genetic predispositions, 5% for environmental exposures, 15% for socioeconomic circumstances and 40% for behavioral patterns, aka lifestyles. Over and above the weight of each of these components, these studies emphasized that, ultimately, "the health fate of each of us is determined by factors acting not mostly in isolation but by our experience where domains interconnect" (McGinnis et al., 2002, p. 83). Thus, while it is undeniable that the creation and consolidation of healthcare systems has significantly improved the population's general health and, consequently, the chances of survival, it is equally clear that we are dealing here with a nonlinear relationship that can be affected by an infinite number of co-occurrences.

To return to the rankings, choosing indicators that lump together aspects that are only partially linked to the services delivered by healthcare systems is not the only problem, as concentrating on efficiency in analyzing the systems' performance can lead to further distortions. Restricting our attention to the economic aspects alone, in fact, can—depending on the circumstances—result in an under- or over-estimation of the quality of a particular healthcare system: spending can be considered efficient when the costs of delivering services are contained even if service quality is low; conversely, high-quality services may be regarded as insufficiently efficient if they employ costly production factors (Cartabellotta et al., 2018, p. 5), as in the case of the new gene therapies or precision medicine. For any given level of life expectancy, for example, it may be that the systems that are judged to be most efficient are in fact those that have cut their resource investments. This is true of Bloomberg's rating for Italy, which rose from sixth to third place between 2013 and 2014 as a result of deploying fewer resources.

The difficulty in understanding the Italian National Health Service's performance (or at least how it is presented) increases if we consider several other well-known ranking systems that describe the situation in different years. According to the Euro Health Consumer Index (Health Consumer Powerhouse, 2018)—which the GIMBE researchers regard as highly reliable because of its continually updated data, multidimensional indicators and the fact that it includes the point of view of the services' actual and/or potential users, which as we will see in the second chapter is by no means to be taken for granted (Cartabellotta et al., 2018, p. 21)—Italy comes 25th out of 35 European countries.[3] The reason for the low score lies in the fact that the 46 indicators for the index's six sub-disciplines—patient rights and information (26th), waiting times for treatment (20th), outcomes (18th), range and reach of services provided (24th), prevention (11th), pharmaceuticals (26th)[4]—are highly heterogeneous because of the large gap between different areas of the country in terms of available services and their accessibility:

> Italy has the largest internal difference of GDP/capita between regions of any European country; the GDP of the poorest region is only 1/3 of that of Lombardy (the richest). Although in theory the entire healthcare system operates under one central ministry of health, the national Index score of Italy is a mix of Northern Italian and Rome Green scores, and Southern Italian Red scores, resulting in a lot of Yellows.
>
> (Health Consumer Powerhouse, 2018, p. 8)

Yet another ranking is the Healthcare Quality and Access Index, calculated for 195 countries and territories over the period 1990–2015 (GBD 2015 Healthcare Access and Quality Collaborators, 2017). Here, the quality of healthcare systems is approximated by measuring the rates of amenable mortality from 32 disease causes, an indicator that takes 11 universal health coverage interventions into account, and the adequacy of human resources in health services. Principal component analysis was used to create a summary measure, where Italy, with a score of 89 out of 100, placed tenth together with Luxembourg and Japan. Though the researchers maintain that the index value is in line with other indicators of healthcare system performance, it is not easy to understand what the final score depends on, and whether and how the response capacity of the analyzed systems has changed over time.

The final comparative assessment system we will deal with here is the OECD Health Database (OECD, 2017, 2019), whose wealth of information is updated twice a year and serves as the basis for a summary report published every two years. Here—unlike the other ranking systems discussed so far—the data are not summarized in a single index, but permit detailed monitoring of 76 indicators grouped into nine categories.[5] The breadth and range of the information in the database provide valuable insights into areas that might require attention, in a level of detail that is unmatched by other surveys: the health workforce category, for example, indicates not only the number of practicing physicians and nurses per 1,000 people but also the average age of medical personnel which, in the case of Italy, enables us to make useful projections about the need to take timely action to forestall the staffing shortages which will soon arise as a result of retirements in the coming years. The data for each country are then collected in Country Health Profiles that provide an overview of the healthcare system, its strong points and weaknesses and how indicators are changing over time, thus giving a full and up-to-date picture of the country's condition and the transformations it has undergone in recent years (OECD/European Observatory on Health Systems and Policies, 2019).

With the exception of the last monitoring system—which, as we have said, provides more analytic information on trends in each country—the international rankings, and the very different scores they assign to Italy, are not very helpful in giving us an idea of how well the healthcare system works and whether it has changed over the years. This is not just because it is always easy to understand (and in some cases agree with) what each monitoring system has chosen to look at and what its goals might be but also because the sheer number of indicators, the varied sources whereby they are monitored and the many different survey timeframes yield such a vast—and at times confused—amount of information that it is virtually impossible to arrive at a clear picture of what is going on. Even bearing in mind that the links between measurement and assessment tools and the objects they are applied to are not always straightforward, our brief review of Italy's standing in the international rankings raises more questions than it answers about the reasons for choosing the different ranking systems, the goals they were developed to meet, how they are used and their actual ability to give us an under-standing of healthcare systems. What types of discourse accompany the data, and what relationship they have with the system they seek to portray will be our topic in the second chapter. To prepare the ground, the following pages will reconstruct the Italian healthcare situation in an attempt to flesh out our understanding of the mechanisms that separate healthcare systems from their description. In doing so, we will map out Italian healthcare's coordinates and the major changes that have taken place in its ability to meet the population's needs.

Though our attention focuses chiefly on Italy, the country is not the fulcrum of our analysis. However, there are several substantive reasons for concentrating on a specific setting that should be mentioned here. First, with a case study approach, our reflections on the narrative and representations of a phenomenon can be empir-ically grounded, reconstructing its coordinates and specificities. Such an approach also enables us to pinpoint exactly what we are unable to determine on the basis of the rankings we start from and helps us gauge the gap between the goals the healthcare system is designed to meet and what it concretely achieves, bearing in mind the assumptions underlying the system as a prerequisite for understanding its effects. As Paci points out in his discussion of the comparative methods used in historical sociology: "Investigating even a single case can not only generate initial hypotheses, but also put them to the test" (2013, p. 312). Close scrutiny of a case casts light on the deep mechanisms that a particular cultural context brings into play, and that can provide insights into the dynamics at work in other contexts. Culture, as Geertz reminds us, "is a context, something in which they [social events, behaviors, institutions, or processes] can be intelligibly—that is, thickly—described" (1973, p. 14), where a thick description by definition gives us a grasp of the context as well as what goes on in it.

In prospective terms, reconstructing the geography of the healthcare system and its variability across time and place in the Italian case study yields a repertoire of tools that, in periods of uncertainty like the present day, can help in making better informed choices of the route toward maintaining the system's sustainability. Reconstructing the principles and assumptions buoying the system helps us to call its outcomes into question, to remember that the decisions we make today will affect the courses taken in the future and that an alternative is often possible and preferable. Starting for the moment from the idea of a reality we can understand and reconstruct, what is the country we are talking about like? What are its characteristics and how have they changed with time?

2 The state of health of the healthcare system in Italy

In her heartfelt defense of the Italian National Health Service on the occasion of its 40th anniversary, Nerina Dirindin, a former Director General of the Ministry of Health, starts by telling a story:

> Do you remember John Q, the 2002 exposé of the US health system? It's the (true) story of a boy who needs a life-saving operation, a heart transplant, but he's not put on a waiting list because his father's insurance won't cover the enormous cost of the procedure (over 250,000 dollars) and the family can't find the money that the hospital wants in cash. Would you like to live in a country where if your son suddenly needed a heart transplant you might be forced to let him die, even if the medical profession was perfectly able to save him?
>
> (Dirindin, 2018, p. 13)

A situation like John Q's could never happen in a universalist system such as the one we have in Italy, despite the many current uncertainties stemming from overstretched resources. Even systems that do not throw up barriers to access, however, spark criticisms and second guessing and certain types of rhetoric that are particularly recurrent in moments of crisis (Hirshman, 1991). Even before the Covid-19 pandemic, for example, the argument was frequently put forward that equity is a luxury we cannot afford and that these systems are no longer sustainable given that access to increasingly personalized treatments would call for an influx of resources that we simply do not have (Longo & Ricci, 2019). These are arguments that bring us to an aspect we will return to several times in this volume: the idea that the principles underlying what it is believed healthcare systems should focus on and what determines their quality do not spring necessarily from concordant visions or common interests, and that the fact that the interests and outlooks vary so widely accounts, at least to some extent, for the differences discussed in the preceding paragraph in what is felt to require monitoring. The point is that we tend to forget this, and the data often take on a weight that is independent of the procedures for which they were collected. Clearly, putting a premium on economic sustainability means turning a favorable eye on choices that dictate cost curbs and put ceilings on expenditure, rewarding parsimony. By contrast, putting a premium on the ability to meet needs and cope with their variability and the inclusive nature of the system presupposes taking a somewhat different perspective, concentrating for instance on the effectiveness of treatment, on patient satisfaction, on healthcare providers' working conditions. In this latter case—as regards treatment outcomes, for example—the results are far more difficult to measure. In this connection, Vineis and Carpi argue that in order to be able to estimate the effectiveness of a treatment it is necessary to be familiar with many details: whether more than one physician agreed on how the clinical tests should be interpreted, if it can be ruled out that different outcomes may depend on factors extraneous to the treatment, like the case itself or its severity, or again, whether physicians and patients followed the protocol appropriately. They conclude that:

> For most medical interventions, at least one of the answers to the preceding questions is still lacking. And for some interventions, none of these questions has been answered.
>
> (Vineis & Capri, 1994, p. 17)

At this point it ought to be clear enough that whether or not a particular system is judged favorably does not depend so much on its inherent nature, but on where an observer decides to look, and on what whoever has the power to do the looking considers valuable, deserving to be retained or, conversely, ripe for change. If what aspects of reality are to be valued is not intrinsic in "things" but constructed in the relationship between actors (Boltanski & Thévenot, 1991; Stark, 2011), the question becomes more political than technical or methodological and calls for a more circumstantiated vision of how the healthcare system works, how equilibrium is reached between the actors involved and the public discourses, and how choices and their outcomes become visible and are justified.

2.1 Principles and transformations of the Italian healthcare system

The Italian National Health System was established a little over 40 years ago by Law 833 of 1978. Though the right to health is enshrined in Article 32 of the Italian Constitution[6]—the only right that the Constitution recognizes as fundamental— the route to a system whereby this right could be applied was long and tortuous, and years went by before the principles on which it is based could be translated into practice. Before 1978, the Italian healthcare system featured three tiers, with wide gaps in coverage between people enrolled in work-related mutual health insurance funds who could thus benefit from higher-quality treatment, those who had to pay for healthcare out of their own pocket, and the "poor" who, lacking in means, were assisted by charitable institutions. In the 1970s, frequent harsh criticism was leveled against the cavalier attitude toward patients' conditions and the state of the often-dilapidated facilities provided to them. An emblematic example of these criticisms was given to us by Gigi Ghirotti, a journalist with the national newspaper *La Stampa*. Diagnosed with life-threatening cancer, Ghirotti decided to face hospitalization without benefiting from the coverage he would have been entitled to because of his profession. Ghirotti's harrowing report on his experience in "the tunnel of illness", aired in 1973 by what was then Italy's only television broadcaster a few short months before Ghirotti's death, raised a furor through its denunciation of the woeful state of Italian healthcare and the obstacles that stand in the way of acceptance for any public debate that includes the patients' perspective in assessing the system's quality.

At the time, the Italian population faced conditions that compared very unfavorably with the rest of Europe from the very beginning of life:

> In Italy, more than 20 newborns died out of every 1000 live births (as against slightly over 9 in France and Sweden) and 30 out of every 1000 children died before their first birthday, versus 10 in Sweden or 15 in France. A catastrophe.
> (Ricciardi, 2019, p. 17)

With the establishment of the National Health Service, the situation changed radically:

> Ensuring that mothers can give birth safely and free of charge in well-equipped wards with skilled personnel has brought these numbers down to an incredible extent. Today, we are second only to Sweden in Europe in terms of maternal/ infant indicators: our neonatal mortality rate is now 2.1 per 1000 versus 1.3 in Finland, and the infant mortality rate is 2.8 against 1.9 per 1000 in Scandinavia.
> (Ricciardi, 2019, p. 17)

Slowly and by no means unopposed, the principles that had been laid down almost 30 years earlier in the Constitution became the pillars of Italy's new healthcare structure. Health now stands at the nexus of individual rights, collective rights and social rights. The idea thus takes hold that (a) health services must be guaranteed for everyone, regardless of individual and social condition or income (the principle of universality); (b) for any given need, everyone has the right to the same services (the principle of equality) and (c) healthcare should not be concentrated only on disease but should be concerned with the person as a whole the (principle of globality) (Zagrebelsky, 2020). The system is financed by general taxation or in other words by the progressive taxes paid by Italian citizens on the basis of the principle that those who have higher incomes pay more taxes, and that the right to healthcare, which is guaranteed to everyone within the country's borders, must depend only on need and not on individual or household finances. The model thus assumes (and hopes) that a redistribution of risks is possible whereby "those who can afford it pay for those in need" (Dirindin, 2018, p. 16) and, since no one can predict what health problems they or their family members will be confronted with (the philosopher John Rawls' *veil of ignorance*, 1971) and thus what costs they will have to bear, the model enables everyone (independently of the resources at their disposal) to face illnesses "so costly that no one could afford the expenses on their own" (Dirindin, 2018, p. 17). Such a division of risk would not be possible with insurance-based systems, since insurance companies are profit-seeking organizations, and policy premiums are thus higher precisely for the people who are at the greatest risk of falling ill. In addition, insurance coverage does not establish a right to healthcare (and thus does not mean that healthcare can in fact be accessed), so we often find that insurers refuse to issue policies to the people who are in the greatest need. The differences between the two types of system are still very substantial: to give an idea of the scale of the issue, Ministry of Health data indicate that each year around 5% of the Italian population receives treatment that is so costly that no one could possibly afford it (and that insurance companies would not reimburse). By way of example, it should be pointed out that in 2016 the National Health Service delivered some 72,000 high-cost procedures (including heart valve surgery, bone marrow and liver transplants and intensive care for severely premature babies) at rates ranging from 20,000 to 63,000 euros (see Ministry of Health, 2016, as cited in Dirindin, 2018, p. 15).

The amazing changes brought about by the National Health Service's entry on the scene would appear to justify Italy's high standing in some of the international classifications discussed in the preceding section, and in fact the service has logged many positive achievements over the years, though they have often been underestimated. While healthcare expenditure as a percentage of GDP is essentially identical to the OECD average (8.9% in 2018 versus 8.8%), the gap with respect to other countries widens if we consider per capita spending (3,542 dollars as against the OECD average of 3,807). The public component of per capita healthcare expenditure (2,622 dollars as against the OECD average of 2,868) is very far from that of countries like Germany and Norway (around 5,000 dollars per capita), and even France and the United Kingdom (Cartabellotta et al., 2019a, p. 76). Even though it can rely on fewer public resources, there are many signs that the Italian system's ability to handle serious illnesses is above the European average, as witnessed by the five-year survival rate for diseases such as lung, prostate, colon and breast cancers, or by the even lower mortality rates for acute myocardial infarction (OECD/European Observatory on Health Systems and Policies, 2019, as cited in Gabriele, 2019, p. 15).

In this case, the data seem to have an undeniable informational value (to which we will return in the second chapter), but this is only part of the story, and the overall picture is naturally richer and moved by dynamics that are more complex than the little information we have mentioned would allow us to glimpse. Not only is the situation of any given healthcare system inevitably more intricate, making it difficult to arrive at a description that can be regarded as objective, but the outcomes of policies (not just Italian policies, and not just healthcare policies) are never the result of a straightforward transposition of the objectives set out on paper. Bearing these caveats in mind, what, today, are the characteristics of the Italian National Health Service, and what has become of the principles that inspired it? According to the experts at the Italian National Institute of Health, the healthcare system model that has developed over the years has changed in ways that threaten to undercut the principles on which it was founded:

> This model held until the Nineties, when lawmakers, faced with the ever more impellent need to cut public spending, renewed their efforts to reduce the range of free services, translating the right to healthcare into a right that— in actual practice—hinged on beneficiary co-pays.
>
> (Celotto, 2018, p. xiii)

Substantive changes in the National Health Service's general approach were brought about by a number of reforms that gradually shifted responsibility for defining and implementing its underlying principles. In 2001, following a partial constitutional reform,[7] the legislature intervened in the existing relationship between the central and regional governments, moving healthcare into the so-called sphere of concurrent competence by establishing that "in the subject matters covered by concurring legislation legislative powers are vested in the Regions, except for the determination of the fundamental principles, which are laid down in State legislation" (Article 117). The state continues to have exclusive competence (Article 117, indent 2) for determining the basic level of benefits relating to civil and social entitlements that each region is required to guarantee, which are then monitored by the central government. For healthcare, this has involved establishing Essential Levels of Care[8] (ELCs) and specifying the activities and services they entail, those that are not included, and those that the National Health Service can deliver only under special circumstances.

Twenty-one regional health care services were thus set up which took the place of the national service. Though the reform was intended to ensure that the specific individual and collective healthcare needs in each region could be more effectively met, it led to wide disparities in organizational approaches and service delivery, thus making it difficult for the central government to perform its coordination and monitoring functions. It must be emphasized here that when systems become increasingly heterogeneous, attempts to show their average trends in synthetic form will always be substantially inadequate for purposes of description and/or comparison. Before turning to the reasons that might in any case justify the use of the highly synthetic measures at the basis of the rankings (see Chapter 2), a few words are in order concerning the changes that have affected the National

Health Service over the years and the aspects that risk eroding its underlying assumptions.

3 Crises and fragility of the Italian National Health Service

A system like Italy's, which is financed chiefly through general tax revenues, is inevitably more vulnerable to the effects of financial crises such as the one that swept the world in 2007:

> The countries that paid, and are still paying, the highest price were those with Beveridge healthcare systems, or in other words with a national health service. The collapse of these countries' finances slashed their tax revenues, which in turn led to cuts in the healthcare sector and thus to a reduction in the services provided, pay freezes, increased staff attrition, and lower rates of technological investment.
>
> (Ricciardi, 2019, p. 14)

This had dire consequences for the Southern European countries. In the case of Italy, the repercussions continued to make themselves felt in the following years: "industrial production down by 25%, gross domestic product down by 10%, record unemployment, buying power at 1994 levels" (Ricciardi, 2019, p. 15). In a situation like Italy's, where the public resources earmarked for the National Health Service are lower than those in other European countries, the economic crisis brings out all the system's fragilities, undermining its stability or, at the very least, mortgaging its future. And this is the grim picture that preceded the Covid-19 explosion and was to make dealing with the pandemic even more complicated. In the decade from 2010 to 2019, the average annual increase in public funding for the National Health Service, at 0.9%, was below the average annual inflation rate of 1.7%: not even enough to maintain constant buying power. Available resources dropped by a total of some 37 billion euros, including 25 in the first five years of the decade as a result of planned budget cuts, and 12 between 2015 and 2019 in order to meet government funding goals, once again by slashing the amounts that had originally been earmarked for healthcare (Cartabellotta et al., 2019b, p. 11). This accentuated the organizational and planning difficulties. Spending on staff was particularly hard-hit, with a reduction in absolute terms of almost 2 billion euros between 2010 and 2018 (Gabriele, 2019). Attrition, or in other words the policy of not replacing retiring employees, resulted in a gradually shrinking workforce, and an increase in the average age of physicians and in the number of Italian residents served by each primary care physician.[9] The condition of medical and nursing personnel was one of the major problems identified by the Parliamentary Budget Office's analysis of the National Health Service, not just because of the particularly sharp drop in the number of nurses, but also because working hours have lengthened well beyond those contemplated by EU regulations,[10] which has worsened working conditions on the whole and increased the risk of burnout (Gabriele, 2019, pp. 25–26).

Looking at a broader timeframe, the number of hospital beds has dropped steadily since the 1980s—as entire hospitals or wards have been closed, and the capacity of those that are still in operation has been reduced. In addition, inpatients' average length of stay for any given disease or procedure has been nearly halved, going from nearly 13 days in the early 1980s to today's 7 (Buzzi & Mozzetta, 2018, p. 3). Hospital beds have dropped from 3.9 per 1,000 population in 2007 to 3.2 in 2017, while the European average has risen from 5.7 to 5 (Gabriele, 2019, p. 23). These figures not only are indicative of the deep-seated changes that have affected Italian healthcare and its organization in recent decades but also show that the meaning of the indicators that purport to describe them is not to be taken for granted. Does dehospitalization mean less ability to meet the population's health needs or better and more innovative ways to provide care? Reaching a consensus about the meaning of measures and the processes they describe, which can be diametrically opposed depending on who uses them and where they are used, is far from automatic.

A good example comes from the changes that have taken place in psychiatric care. The movement that led to the law that closed Italy's mental hospitals (Law 180/78) in the same year that the National Health Service was established took deinstitutionalizing psychiatric patients and reintegrating them in the community as one of its driving principles. As a result of this law, mental hospital beds dropped from almost 68,000 in 1981 to 5,600 in 2016 (Gabriele, 2019, p. 10). In this case, dehospitalization was touted as an alternative model for dealing with mental distress. It was thus the result, not of a cutback in resources, but of a wager that an alternative system could be set up that would be more effective from the clinical and social standpoints. The idea was that these two aspects were closely linked and that, to improve the clinical situation, it was also necessary to consider the patients' interaction with society and thus throw open the places of reclusion that had spawned so many illnesses.

Taking an entirely different perspective, many planning documents see dehospitalization as a process that makes it possible to achieve significant savings and rationalize healthcare provision, and agree that the future of healthcare must move away from hospital services for organizational as well as economic reasons, for example, by closing smaller and less viable hospitals (Longo & Ricci, 2019). It is also argued that reducing the number of beds could improve care pathways by leading to a system that no longer centers on the hospital, but opens out onto a wider area through an approach that not only flanks normal inpatient and outpatient care but also enables the public to turn to local health centers or various types of home health service where available (Ibidem, p. 24). But this perspective is not the only one that can be taken in interpreting the issue. A certain ambivalence stems from the multiple meanings attached to the term dehospitalization, which range from reducing hospital stays to shifting from ordinary inpatient care to day hospital treatment, as well as to moving services provided during hospital stays to outpatient facilities, the home, or elsewhere (Zocchetti & Cislaghi, 2011).

Obvious as it may seem, it is all too easy to forget that, depending on which of these meanings is considered, the data will differ, and not all of them will be equally easy to document. But in addition to questions of measurement, whether dehospitalization processes are seen as positive or negative might not depend on abstract qualities, but on how the different organizational levels that must deal with them are connected to each other: shortening hospital stays, for instance, could be regarded as a good thing if adequate forms of home care enable patients to continue treatment after being discharged. It would be quite another matter if local services are inadequate or lacking and patients who had had surgery only a few days before were obliged to shuttle back and forth from home to hospital for daily medication or therapy.

According to the Parliamentary Budget Office, the problem of achieving integration between local and hospital services—so that some proportion of healthcare can be handled at the district level—is one of the thorniest issues facing the National Health Service:

> Italy has undoubtedly scaled back hospital services but this does not appear to have been matched by a sufficient reinforcement of the facilities available locally or of their integration, especially in certain regions.
>
> (Gabriele, 2019, p. 21)

Though scaling back hospital services could be positive from the standpoint of organizational appropriateness, not just for cost reasons, but also—to cite a single example—as a way of preventing the spread of nosocomial infections, patients and caregivers would be justified in taking another view. Indeed, they frequently complain that the shortage of beds and faster discharges shift the burden of care that was formerly borne by the hospital onto family members or paid help, sending patients home "quicker but sicker" (Qian et al., 2011). As we will see, however, what we have just described is not the only area where meanings are blurred.

3.1 Shuttling between public and private provision

The changes in healthcare spending, in particular in the balance between public and private and inpatient co-pays and other out-of-pocket payments, add further reasons to be cautious about synthetic indicators' ability to offer a grounded description of the system's characteristics and the outcomes of these changes. Over the years, the Italian National Health Service has taken a particular form that places it in the category of predominantly public mixed systems. On the supply side, accredited private providers deliver a sizable share of healthcare services under contract with the national system, which means that part of the *public* expenditure is used to pay *private* providers of the services available to Italy's residents (Vineis & Capri, 1994). Over and above any debate about the advantages that might accrue or the criticisms that could be leveled against having private actors in the healthcare system, the complexity of the public/private mix in healthcare provision and financing makes monitoring trends far from easy. And how the out-of-pocket payments required of large swaths of the population have changed over time makes the picture even more complicated. Starting in the 1990s, several reform processes introduced and gradually increased user charges for healthcare services. In particular, Legislative Decree 502/92 established three financing channels: public funding, which guarantees only the Essential Levels of Care (ELCs); collective complementary healthcare, which is intended to cover services that are not included in the ELC package through private insurance funds and policies; and individual healthcare, which consists of taking out voluntary health insurance policies or direct purchases of tax-deductible healthcare goods and services. According to the most recent available data, Italy's private healthcare expenditure in 2017 accounted for 27% of the total, most of which (86%) consisted of out-of-pocket expenses in the form of user cost-sharing (as will be discussed later) and payments for private services such as dental care (Cartabellotta et al., 2019a, p. 15). At an estimated 23.5% of total spending, out-of-pocket payments in Italy are quite high compared to France (9.4%) and the average for countries with a public national health service (19.3%) (Armeni et al., 2019). According to the WHO (2010), this is a major concern, as higher direct out-of-pocket payments increase the risk of impoverishment. The WHO thus establishes a threshold value:

> when direct payments rise above 20% of total health expenditure, households coping with illness face financial catastrophe.
>
> (Giarelli, 2014, p. 354)

In Italy, user cost-sharing—rising slowly but steadily in recent years—applies to a range of services that has seen a series of piecemeal additions since 1993 (Fenech & Panfili, 2013). In that year, Law 537/1993 introduced the so-called "ticket", a form of co-pay levied on specialist visits, diagnostic procedures and laboratory tests. Specific exemptions from cost-sharing are envisaged for the services provided for severe illnesses and chronic conditions (DM 329/99), while the services included in the ELC package are fully covered to prevent patients' condition from deteriorating (DM 279/2001). Further types of cost-sharing include a 25 euro charge for inappropriate use of emergency services which do not result in hospital admission, and an additional 10 euro co-pay—the so-called "super ticket"—on top of the standard co-payment for specialist visits.[11] Two aspects of this complex situation should be emphasized: the first is the lack of uniformity in the regions' cost-sharing decisions. In the case of the "super ticket", for example, some regional healthcare systems have decided not to apply it. Of the regions that have adopted the measure, some levy the fixed 10 euro charge; others calculate a charge proportionate to the user's income, and others again use a percentage of the cost of the service (Ibidem, 132). Though these are obviously legitimate decisions, they create further disparities between residents of different parts of the country. The second aspect concerns an indirect repercussion of the increase in the costs users must bear to access public services. Though the stated objective of greater cost-sharing was to boost public revenues, its effect has been to tip the unsteady public/private balance further in favor of private providers, who as we have said are in any case paid out of the public purse for services offered under contract:

> A large proportion of laboratory checks, blood tests for example, are delivered at very low unit prices: an enormous number of tests cost less than 2 euros, and a non-exempt user is required to pay only up to a maximum ceiling of 36.15 euros. Thus, to give an example, a prescription for eight blood tests (each costing 2 euros) will involve, if the user goes to the public healthcare service, an outlay of 26 euros (16 euros for the eight tests plus 10 for the super ticket). The same tests at a private center will cost 16 euros, because the charge for the super ticket does not apply if the National Health Service is not used.
>
> (Dirindin, 2018, p. 49)

The consequences can be significant: with the "progressive withdrawal of public healthcare from specialist outpatient services" and the corresponding increase of private provision in a particularly lucrative area, the proliferation of small laboratories can make them more difficult to monitor and encourage less rigorous means of control. It can then lead to a "willful neglect of the principle of appropriateness", given that the private provider might have no incentive to limit unneeded but remunerative diagnostic procedures. It could also increase the number of well-heeled taxpayers seeking to opt out of the National Health Service and turn to forms of private healthcare (Dirindin, 2018, p. 50).

Another factor that tends to make users move from public to private providers is the increase in waiting times, especially for diagnostic services and specialist visits. Waiting times are such a problem that the question has been addressed over the years by a number of ad hoc surveys and specific legislation[12] as well as by nationwide planning documents to formulate policies for reducing them, as in the case of the National Waiting List Management Plan (PNGLA) for 2019–2021. The Management Plan is tasked with drawing up a full list of inpatient and outpatient specialist services and assigning a priority class to each, which establishes the maximum number of days within which the services must be provided. By way of example, according to the Parliamentary Budget Office:

> in 2017, average waiting times were over 27 days for breast cancer, 53 for prostate cancer, 119 for a tonsillectomy, 90 for inguinal hernia. According to data published by the Italian Court of Auditors (2019), a nationwide survey found that in 2018 the percentage of priority class B services that were effectively provided within the guaranteed 10 days oscillated between 78 and 87 per cent for eight services, while the percentage of class D services—which are guaranteed to take place within 30 days for visits and 60 days for diagnostic procedures—that in fact met targets ranged from 68 to 95 per cent. In most (7 out of 8) of the most urgent cases, these figures were worse than in the previous year.
>
> (Gabriele, 2019, p. 31)

Though the central government's three-year plans have laid down a significant number of requirements for the regions, complete up-to-date data are still not available for all regions. Within 60 days of the approval of the National Waiting List Management Plan, each regional government should have adopted its own Regional Management Plan. As of May 2019, 12 out of 21 regional systems had still not done so, and for the remaining nine, the level of information—needed both for regional planning purposes and to deal with demand from patients and the public—varied widely (Cartabellotta et al., 2019c, p. 11). The lack of clear, accessible information not only complicates efforts to monitor trends, it also produces a mechanism similar to the one we described for diagnostic procedures.

For the individual, higher co-pays and the difficulty in obtaining services within a reasonable period of time make it more rational to turn to accredited private facilities or to the *intra-moenia* framework,[13] whereby National Health Service physicians can take privately paying patients at public facilities outside normal hospital working hours. Parenthetically, it should be noted that the opportunity to be treated by the same physicians at the same facilities but with markedly shorter waiting time by paying for services directly is an issue that has roiled the healthcare debate for years. A number of patients' advocacy groups and physicians' associations have taken up warring stances, but for the moment no common ground has been found (D'Angelo, 2018).

Clearly, the dynamics we have outlined here have brought about a substantive change in how the system operates and undercut the cardinal principle of universality on which the Italian National Health Service had long been based. It is equally possible that synthetic indicators that seek to describe the system's operation are not capable of investigating its dynamics in detail, thus contributing to drawing a picture that has very little to do with what the system is really like.

3.2 Geographical disparities and possible repercussions on the healthcare system

We have mentioned the redistributive intentions behind the birth of the National Health Service in the 1970s. This idea did not spring only from an awareness that class differences have a significant impact on the population's living conditions and health but also arose out of the legislator's desire to close the yawning gap between different parts of the country. The connection between place of residence and the population's health has been extensively investigated in the field of health geography (Jivraj et al., 2019) and in studies of health inequalities and their determinants (Mirisola et al., 2017). For example, several studies have found that inequalities in life expectancy can be produced on a very small geographical scale, pointing to the so-called "neighborhood effect", whereby living in disadvantaged areas can have long-term repercussions on health in proportion to the duration of residence. On the base of the findings of a longitudinal study conducted in Torino, a northern Italian city of around 1 million inhabitants, it has been estimated that "a man who moves across the city, from the upper middle class, high-income hills overlooking Torino to the low-income working class neighborhoods on the northwestern outskirts will see his life expectancy drop by six months for every kilometer" (Costa et al., 2017, reported in Mirisola et al., 2017, p. 8).

In Italy, the data show that the geographical inequalities between regions have increased over time. This is one of the most severe problems that the country's healthcare organization must deal with to avoid the risk of the so-called "inverse care law", which states that those who are most in need of healthcare are often the least likely to receive it (Mirisola et al., 2017, p. 40).

Over the years, a variety of measures have been deployed to increase the regional healthcare systems' accountability for reducing the inequalities and reaching the minimum standards set for each area. For example, a portion of the central government's funding for the regions was pegged to a series of requirements to be met by the regional governments. Regions that failed to perform as expected or ran excessive deficits were obliged to adopt the so-called Financial Recovery Plans which set limits on spending and monitored progress toward rectifying the situation by a specified deadline. Failure to show improvement triggered tightened sanctions, culminating in curbs on the region's autonomy and the appointment of a special government commissioner. Nine (out of 20) regions were required to adopt Financial Recovery Plans between 2007 and 2010, and five were put under the administration of a special commissioner. These were the years of the global crisis and in several southern regions—already in a far weaker condition than their northern counterparts—sanctions included a complete hiring freeze or blocked nonessential spending for lengthy periods. Though this helped put the regions' budgets on a somewhat sounder footing, it also worsened regional disparities and proved detrimental to the condition of patients in many areas. Once again, national averages are of little use in describing the broad range of healthcare conditions in Italy and how they vary from region to region. We have already spoken of the general reduction in healthcare staffing, but this takes on an entirely different complexion if we compare the regions that had to implement a recovery plan with those that did not:

> Between 2008 and 2017, the regions under standard recovery plans saw the number of physicians drop by 18 percent and nurses by 11, while the number of non-medical managers fell by 23 percent and the remaining non-management personnel by around 20 percent. The regions with light recovery plans made significant cuts in non-medical management staff (14 percent) and other non-management personnel (8 percent), and smaller cuts in physicians and nurses (3 and 2 percent respectively). In the regions that did not have to adopt a recovery plan, the number of physicians remained stable, while there was a limited reduction in other staff.
>
> (Gabriele, 2019, p. 21)

Spurred by the need to get the deficit under control, the staff cuts made existing disparities worse in some regions, and healthcare federalism, which was supposed to reduce these disparities, in fact contributed to making them larger. This situation is illustrated schematically in Figure 1.1. According to the Parliamentary Budget Office, the main differences are exemplified by three categories. The grey line in the radar chart represents interregional patient mobility or, in other words, movements by patients who are unable to find treatment in their own region. The need to seek treatment in places that are often very far from home creates obvious difficulties for patients and their families as they face the heavy human and economic costs of lengthy hospital stays. The regions that attract patients are chiefly those in the Center-North (Lombardia, Veneto and Emilia Romagna in particular), whose greater wealth is reflected in higher levels of healthcare resources. Patient mobility is a complex phenomenon that exacerbates the inequalities between different parts of the country, as it means further transfers of funds from the regions with high patient outflows (who are required to pay for their residents' treatment even if it takes place in other regions) toward those with high inflows:

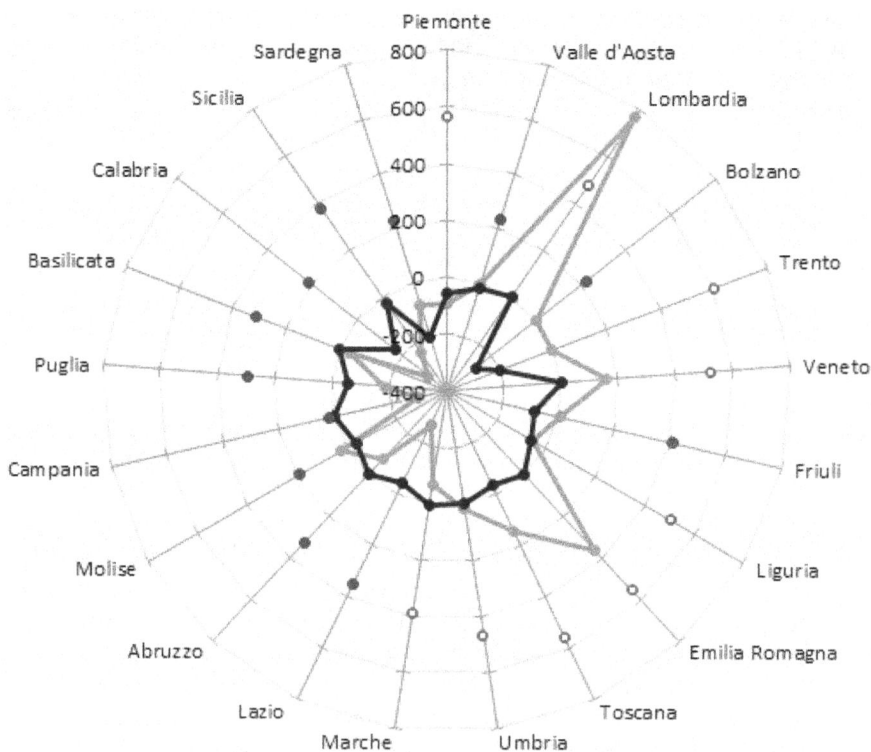

Figure 1.1 Differences between Italy's regional healthcare systems (data on patient mobility and operating results in millions of euros in 2018; satisfactory and unsatisfactory performance in Essential Levels of Care in 2016)

Source: Parliamentary Budget Office, calculations based on data from the State General Accounting Department, Gabriele, 2019, p. 34.

Thus, the former [i.e., the regions with high patient outflows], in addition to having fewer resources to invest in their own healthcare systems, thus contribute both to financing the healthcare services (and ultimately the economic system) of the latter regions, and to overcrowding them.

(Gabriele, 2019, p. 33)

Going back to Figure 1.1, the black line represents operating results, i.e., the regional healthcare systems' ability to balance their budgets and implement the cost-curbing measures called for by the recovery plans. Lastly, the dots indicate the adequacy of services in 2016, measured on the basis of synthetic indicators for prevention, hospital care and district care: the circled dots identify the regions that performed satisfactorily, scoring at least 60 out of the 100 points envisaged for the indicator, while the black dots indicate the regions with sub-par performance.

Even without going into the details of these differences, the figure makes it clear that there are still major disparities in performance levels that can have significant effects on health inequalities in Italy's regions and accentuate the long-standing social and economic gap that separates them.

4 Conclusions

Our description of Italy's healthcare has illustrated how complex systems are inevitably subject to changes over time that shift their coordinates. It should now be sufficiently clear just how difficult it is to produce synthetic assessments of healthcare efforts that can monitor their characteristics and how they change. We have seen that there are many different reasons for this: demonstrating that treatments are effective and developing suitable indicators for measuring them is a complex operation that tends to fall back on data about the process (the number of services provided, for example) rather than about outcomes (whether the services worked or not) (Vineis & Capri, 1994); the lack of a widespread data culture (or a culture of using data purposively) means that even the information that in theory could be available is neither precise, complete nor up-to-date; indicators are used (as in the case of life expectancy) which depend only partially on healthcare systems' performance; national averages are used even for contexts that are known to be heterogeneous; and indicators averaged over long periods of time are used, which does not help in understanding whether the policies that have been introduced have improved the situation and what changes have taken place. Because of these innumerable complications, the ability of ranking systems to describe the nature of healthcare systems and compare them would appear to be unsatisfactory in many respects. Why then, despite the fact that they have been found to be inadequate in many cases, are ranking systems so highly regarded? What is the nature of information in the field of healthcare, and how is this information linked to the policies put in place? In the next chapter, our attention will shift from healthcare systems and their measurement to the nature of the information that circulates and the many different objectives that contribute to defining their coordinates.

Notes

1 In healthcare, efficiency refers to the goal of obtaining the maximum benefit from the resources deployed. Economically speaking, a distinction is usually made between two dimensions of efficiency: "technical efficiency seeks to provide maximum service quality at the lowest cost; allocative efficiency refers to how available resources are used to obtain the optimal mix of services and outputs which maximizes health benefits" (Cartabellotta, 2009, p. 4). The former dimension is commonly employed, given the difficulty of measuring the latter.

2 Effectiveness is the ability of an action to achieve the desired effects. It is gauged through outcomes research, which "identifies the extent of the benefits obtained by healthcare" (Cartabellotta, 2009, p. 4) and must take account "of the reliability and completeness of information systems, and of other health determinants such as genetic and environmental factors, culture and socioeconomic conditions" (Ibidem).

3 In addition to the 28 EU member states, the classification includes Norway, Switzerland, Republic of Macedonia, Iceland, Serbia, Montenegro and Bosnia-Herzegovina.

4 For each sub-discipline, Italy's position in the ranking is shown in parentheses.

5 The nine categories (health status, risk factors for health, access to care, quality and outcomes of care, health expenditure, health workforce, health care activities, pharmaceutical sector, aging and long-term care) and their 76 indicators refer to the 35 OECD member countries. For some of the indicators, Brazil, People's Republic of China, Colombia, Costa Rica, India, Indonesia, Lithuania, Russia and South Africa.

6 Article 32 of the Constitution—promulgated in December 1947—states:

> The Republic safeguards health as a fundamental right of the individual and as a collective interest, and guarantees free medical care to the indigent. No one may be obliged to undergo any health treatment except under the provisions of the law. The law may not under any circumstances violate the limits imposed by respect for the human person.

7 Constitutional Law No. 3 of October 18, 2001.

8 The Decree of the President of the Council of Ministers of November 29, 2001, "Essential Levels of Care" was amended by the Decree of January 12, 2017.

9 The number of primary care physicians per 10,000 inhabitants went from almost 11 to fewer than 9 in 2013, the last year for which data are available (Buzzi & Mozzetta, 2018, p. 4).

10 Since 2015, on the basis of Law 161/2014, the disapplication of EU legislation is no longer permitted, and several measures have been implemented to reorganize shifts and jobs.

11 The "super ticket" was abolished by the annual Budget Act at the end of 2019.

12 The question of waiting lists was addressed in particular by Laws 724/1994 and 266/2005. The latest 2019–2021 National Waiting List Management Plan was approved on February 21, 2019, by the Conference on the Relationships between central government, the regions and the self-governing provinces, and the regions should have transposed it into their own regional plans within 60 days.

13 The *intra-moenia* framework for intramural private practice enables physicians employed at a hospital to provide services outside their normal working hours using the hospital's outpatient and diagnostic facilities, charging the patient a fee. The physician is required to issue a regular invoice, and the fee, like all medical expenses, is tax deductible. The services are generally those that the physicians in question are required to provide during their normal work on the hospital staff under the terms of their employment contract with the National Health Service. Services provided under the *intra-moenia* framework ensure that patients are able to choose the physician attending them (Ministry of Health, 2013).

References

Armeni, P., Bertolani, A., Borsoi, L., & Costa, F. (2019). *La spesa sanitaria: composizione ed evoluzione*. In *Rapporto OASI 2019. Osservatorio sulle Aziende e sul Sistema sanitario Italiano: 99–152*. CERGAS—Bocconi. www.cergas.unibocconi.eu/wps/wcm/connect/4c40095a-2ca4-4c9f-828c-385db9e4d9db/Cap3OASI_2019.pdf?MOD=AJPE RES&CVID=mWPG7t3.

Bloomberg. (2014). *Most Efficient Health Care 2014: Countries*. www.bloomberg.com/graphics/best-and-worst/#mostefficient-health-care-2014-countries.

Boltanski, L., & Thévenot, L. (1991). *De la justification. Les économies de la grandeur*. Paris: Édition Gallimard. English translation by Catherine Porter (2006), *On Justification. Economies of Worth*. Princeton University Press.

Buzzi, N., & Mozzetta, I. (Eds.). (2018). *SSN40. Rapporto Sanità 2018.40 anni del Servizio Sanitario Nazionale*. Nebo Ricerche PA. https://programmazionesanitaria.it/_progsan/2018/SSN40-Rapporto.pdf.

Cartabellotta, A. (2009). La valutazione multidimensionale della qualità assistenziale. L'efficienza continua a oscurare gli indicatori di clinical governance? *GIMBEnews, 3*, 4–5. www.evidence.it/articolodettaglio/209/it/80/la-valutazione-multidimensionale-della-qualit%C3%A0-assistenziale-l/articolo.

Cartabellotta, N., Cottafava, E., Luceri, R., & Mosti, M. (2019a). *4° Rapporto sulla sostenibilità del Servizio Sanitario Nazionale*. Bologna: Fondazione GIMBE, June. www.rapportogimbe.it.

Cartabellotta, N., Cottafava, E., Luceri, R., & Mosti, M. (2019b). *Il definanziamento 2010–2019 del Servizio Sanitario Nazionale*. Report Osservatorio GIMBE n. 7/2019. Bologna: Fondazione GIMBE, September. www.gimbe.org/definanziamento-SSN.

Cartabellotta, N., Cottafava, E., Luceri, R., Mosti, M., & Orsi, F. (2018). *Il Servizio Sanitario Nazionale nelle classifiche internazionali*. Report Osservatorio GIMBE, n.4/2018, September. www.gimbe.org/osservatorio/Report_Osservatorio_GIMBE_2018.04_Classifiche_SSN.pdf.

Cartabellotta, N., Gianfredi, V., Luceri, R., Cottafava, E., & Mosti, M. (2019c). *Tempi di attesa: trasparenza di Regioni e Aziende sanitarie*. Report Osservatorio GIMBE n. 4/2019. Bologna: Fondazione GIMBE, September. www.gimbe.org/osservatorio/Report_Osservatorio_GIMBE_2019.04_Liste_attesa.pdf.

Celotto, A. (2018). Breve storia legislativa della sanità in Italia. In Ricciardi, W., Alleva, E., De Castro, P., Giuliano, F., & Salinetti, S. (Eds.), *1978–2018: Forty Years of Science and Public Health. The Voice of the Istituto Superiore di Sanità*. Istituto Superiore di Sanità, ix–xiv. http://old.iss.it/binary/publ/cont/40anni_SSN_scenza_sanitpubblica.pdf.

Costa, G., Demaria, M., Stroscia, M., Zengarini, N., Bianco, S., Ferracin, E., Mamo, C., Melis, G., & Tabasso, M. (2017). La salute nei quartieri: conta di più chi sei o dove vivi? In Costa, G., Stroscia, M., Zengarini, N., & Demaria, M. (Eds.), *40 anni di salute a Torino. Spunti per leggere i bisogni e i risultati delle politiche*. Milano: Inferenze, 68–89.

Court of Auditors. (2019). https://www.corteconti.it/Download?id=8953477e-83b4-46f1-af74-49a18387441f

D'Angelo, F. (2018). Liste di attesa e libera professione, nodi da sciogliere in favore della salute, dalla Lombardia alla Puglia. *Medicina Democratica*. www.medicinademocratica.org/wp/?p=7330.

Dirindin, N. (2018). *E' tutta salute. In difesa della sanità pubblica*. Torino: Edizioni Gruppo Abele.

European Commission's Directorate-General for Economic and Financial Affairs. (2016). *Report on Public Finances in EMU*. Institutional paper 045, December. https://ec.europa.eu/info/sites/info/files/ip045_en_0.pdf.

Fenech, L., & Panfili, A. (2013). L'evoluzione del ticket in Italia. Gli effetti delle politiche sulla spesa sanitaria delle famiglie e prospettive future. *Salute e Territorio, XXXIV*(198), 129–137. www.formas.toscana.it/rivistadellasalute/fileadmin/files/fascicoli/2013/198/FILE_198_intero_w.pdf.

Gabriele, S. (2019). *Lo stato della sanità in Italia*. Focus Tematico 6, Ufficio Parlamentare di Bilancio (UPB), December. www.upbilancio.it/wp-content/uploads/2019/12/Focus_6_2019-sanit%C3%A0.pdf.

GBD 2015 Healthcare Access and Quality Collaborators. (2017). Healthcare Access and Quality Index Based on Mortality from Causes Amenable to Personal Health Care in 195 Countries and Territories, 1990–2015—A Novel Analysis from the Global Burden of Disease Study 2015. *Lancet, 390*, 231–266. https://doi.org/10.1016/S0140-6736(17)30818-8.

Geerz, C. (1973). *The Interpretation of Cultures*. New York: Basic Books.

Giarelli, G. (2014). La copertura sanitaria universale fra retorica e realtà: una prospettiva internazionale. *Politiche Sociali, 3*, 353–372. https://doi.org/10.7389/78431.

Health Consumer Powerhouse. (2018). *Euro Health Consumer Index 2017 Report*. Health Consumer Powerhouse Ltd. https://healthpowerhouse.com/media/EHCI-2017/EHCI-2017-report.pdf www.salute.gov.it/portale/temi/p2_6.jsp?lingua=italiano&id=1237&area=ricoveriOspedalieri&menu=vuoto.

Hirshman, A. (1991). *The Rhetoric of Reaction. Perversity, Futility, Jeopardy*. Cambridge, MA: The Belknap Press of Harvard University Press.

Jivraj, S., Murray, E. T., Norman, P., & Nicholas, O. (2019). The Impact of Life Course Exposures to Neighbourhood Deprivation on Health and Well-Being: A Review of the Long-Term Neighborhood Effects Literature. *European Journal of Public Health*, 1–7. https://doi.org/10.1093/eurpub/ckz153.

Longo, F., & Ricci, A. (2019). *Ridefinire la missione del SSN nell'universo sanitario in espansione: prospettive strategiche per promuovere l'innovazione*. In *Osservatorio sulle Aziende e sul Sistema sanitario Italiano, Rapporto OASI 2019: 1–32*. CERGAS—Bocconi. www.cergas.unibocconi.eu/wps/wcm/connect/282b216d-6392-47b9-9ac7-5efa076d6890/Cap1OASI_2019.pdf?MOD=AJPERES&CVID=mWPFMg0.

McGinnis, J. M., Williams-Russo, P., & Knickman, J. R. (2002). The Case for More Active Policy Attention to Health Promotion, *Health Affairs, 21*(2), 78–93. www.healthaffairs.org/doi/pdf/10.1377/hlthaff.21.2.78.

McKee, M., & Stuckler, D. (2011). The Assault on Universalism: How to Destroy the Welfare State. *British Medical Journal, 343*, d7973. https://doi.org/10.1136/bmj.d7973.

Ministry of Health. (2013). *Intramoenia, la nuova disciplina*. www.salute.gov.it/portale/temi/p2_6.jsp?lingua=italiano&id=3310&area=professioni-sanitarie&menu=intramuraria

Ministry of Health. (2016). *Rapporto Schede Dimissioni Ospedaliere. https://www.salute.gov.it/portale/documentazione/p6_2_2_1.jsp?lingua=italiano&id=2651)*.

Mirisola, C., Ricciardi, G., Bevere, F., & Melazzini, M. (Eds.). (2017). *L'Italia per l'Equità nella Salute*. Ministero della Salute. www.inmp.it/ita/Pubblicazioni/Libri/L-Italia-per-l-equita-nella-salute-Scarica-il-documento-tecnico.

OECD. (2017). *Health at a Glance 2017: OECD Indicators*. Paris: OECD Publishing. www.oecd-ilibrary.org/social-issues-migration-health/health-at-a-glance-2017_health_glance-2017-en.

OECD. (2019). *Health at a Glance 2019: OECD Indicators*. Paris: OECD Publishing. https://doi.org/10.1787/4dd50c09-en.

OECD/European Observatory on Health Systems and Policies. (2019). *Italy: Country Health Profile 2019, State of Health in the EU*. Paris: OECD Publishing—Brussels: European Observatory on Health Systems and Policies. https://doi.org/10.1787/cef1e5cb-en.

Paci, M. (2013). *Lezioni di sociologia storica*. Bologna: Il Mulino. https://doi.org/10.978.8815/314055.

Qian, X., Russell, L. B., Valiyeva, E., & Miller, J. E. (2011). "Quicker and Sicker" Under Medicare's Prospective Payment System for Hospitals: New Evidence on an Old Issue from a National Longitudinal Survey. *Bulletin of Economic Research, 63*(1), 1–27. https://doi.org/10.1111/j.1467-8586.2010.00369.x.

Rawls, J. (1971). *A Theory of Justice*. Harvard: Harvard University Press.

Ricciardi, W. (2019). *La battaglia per la salute*. Bari: Editori Laterza.

Stark, D. (2011). *The Sense of Dissonance. Accounts of Worth in Economic Life*. Princeton: Princeton University Press.

Vineis, P., & Capri, S. (1994). *La salute non è una merce. Efficacia della medicina e politiche sanitarie*. Torino: Bollati Boringhieri.

WHO. (2010). *The World Health Report. Health Systems Financing. The Path to Universal Coverage*. Geneva: World Health Organization. www.who.int/whr/2010/whr10_en.pdf?ua=1.

Zagrebelsky, V. (2020). *Il diritto alla salute al tempo dell'epidemia, Conversazioni ai tempi del Coronavirus, 3 aprile 2020 — Conversazione N.1*. [Audio podcast]. www.carloalberto.org/cca-events/carlo-alberto-on-air/conversazioni-ai-tempi-del-coronavirus/.

Zocchetti, C., & Cislaghi, C. (2011). GRANCHI/Attenzione a come si misura la deospedalizzazione Measuring de-Hospitalization is not an Easy Job: Pay Attention! *Epidemiologia&Prevenzione,35*(1),61–66. www.epiprev.it/rubrica/granchiattenzione-come-si-misura-la-deospedalizzazione.

Chapter 2

Bringing healthcare policies into focus

Measuring, describing, evaluating and choosing

Twenty years have passed since the World Health Organization (WHO) made the first broad-based attempt at worldwide ratings, analyzing the performance of health systems in 191 countries across the globe. Given its significance and scale, this initiative echoed long and loud, particularly in countries that, like Italy, France and Spain, were tapped as the top health system performers. These countries scored higher in the ranking than others—Canada, Germany, Sweden and Denmark, for instance—which are often held up as models of good public healthcare—and higher than the United States, whose system is radically different but could bring far larger expenditures into play. The report was based on five composite indicators:

> Overall level of population health; health inequalities (or disparities) within the population; overall level of health system responsiveness (a combination of *patient satisfaction* and how well the system acts); *distribution of responsiveness with the population (how well people of varying economic status find that they are served by the health system);* and the distribution of the health system's financial burden within the population (who pays the costs).
> (WHO, 2000, as cited in Blendon et al., 2001, p. 11)

Including patients' satisfaction with the quality of the care they received would suggest that the various segments of each country's population to which the indicators referred were consulted. This, however, was not the case: the ratings were based entirely on interviews with public health experts, and the groups in question were in no way involved. Blendon et al. (2001) point out that this choice was explicitly justified at the time in the background papers to the WHO report, which stated that—methodologically speaking—experts are the only ones who can express reliable judgments. It was argued that:

> How well a health system performs is too complex for the general public to understand; it involves basic knowledge of public health issues that are not well understood; and patients' perceptions are too narrow to fully assess a health system.
> (Gakidou et al., 2000, in Blendon et al., 2001, p. 11)

DOI: 10.4324/9780367854515-3

Though the researchers considered experts' opinion of the more technical questions to be essential, Blendon and colleagues doubted that this domain should be left entirely to experts, or that their judgments could help build a consensus picture of the system's quality. Parenthetically, it should be noted that there has been considerable debate on the role of experts in a number of spheres, including that of occupational safety, where an enlarged scientific community—comprising experts, academics, workers, activists and social researchers—is now seen as central in gaining a full knowledge of the processes involved and taking appropriate action to improve working conditions and worker protection (Burawoy, 2005; Re, 2015, as cited in Borghi, 2019, pp. 47–48).

Given, however, that this was not the perspective taken in the WHO report, Blendon and colleagues (2001) decided to test their hypotheses in a subset of 17 countries, determining how consistent the report's findings were with those of other surveys,[1] which tapped public opinion directly. This comparison showed significant differences between the experts' evaluations and those of the public: though Italy was ranked second by the WHO, only 20% of the country's citizens declared themselves satisfied with their healthcare system at the time of the survey. At the other end of the spectrum, Denmark's 16th place in the ranking appeared to have little relationship with the satisfaction expressed by 91% of the population. The differences were even more marked if we look at the views of the more vulnerable populations within the surveyed countries, e.g., the poor and the elderly. In this case, Italy dropped from second place out of 191 countries to 15th out of 17 (Blendon et al., 2001). Nevertheless, the high standing that Italy's healthcare system enjoyed, thanks to its place in the WHO ranking, was long taken for granted:

> This recognition was touted as a source of national pride for over fifteen years, and is still mentioned in institutional documents, despite the fact that the methodologies have been harshly criticized and the information dates back to 1997. Considering that the WHO never intended the World Health Report to be an assessment of healthcare systems' performance, this "position" of the National Health Service should no longer be cited, except for historical reasons.
>
> (Cartabellotta et al., 2018, pp. 8–9)

It is little short of amazing to note that even though the WHO ranking has been widely criticized (Cooley & Snyder, 2015) and many years have gone by since the situation that the data described, many people continue to consider it—and not only in Italy—as one of the most complete in terms of the methodology's reproducibility and transparency (Schütte et al., 2018). That certain assumptions have persisted despite the empirical evidence which has cast doubt on their basis in fact and their consequences in terms of choices made from premises that would seem to be ambiguous or have been proven false does not appear to have limited the report's circulation or references to its findings. How can we explain the paradox of such dissimilar judgments about the same ranking system? Why does it continue to be used despite the evidence of its shortcomings? These questions and the more general issue of the relationship between information and practices in healthcare will be addressed in the following pages.

1 What we measure, how we measure it and why and how the world changes as a result

The discussion about the role assigned to experts is an example of the ambivalences we encounter whenever we are dealing—as in the case of the right to health—with aspects that are complex and central to our lives as individuals and members of a community. It might seem unnecessary to explain what we think ought to be measured in a certain context, or how and why we intend to measure it and who will be delegated to do so, and that a commonsense answer like "we measure what's important" might seem to be enough. In fact, collecting information and making it accessible is the main justification advanced for the effort behind ranking systems.

As regards organizational analysis and ranking systems' repercussions, a recent review of the literature published between 2010 and 2018 in the major international journals of management, sociology, education and law points to contributing information as one of the three principal perspectives on ranking systems and their use (Rindova et al., 2018). The "information intermediation perspective" sees ranking systems essentially as tools needed to compensate for the inevitable information asymmetries between the actors involved, both by publicly circulating information that is usually available to few people and thus making it accessible to a broader public and by decoding this information so that it is comprehensible to stakeholders. Recognizing that information is central, the studies considered in the review assign great importance to its quality and to the effectiveness of the dimensions and indicators used in describing the actual situation of the organizations considered. The underlying idea is that it is possible to produce more complete, understandable pictures of the organizations' priorities and that the circulation of information can, by its very nature, promote consensus in the resulting decisions.

The example of the WHO ranking system, however, should have made it clear enough that things are in reality less obvious. The variability of the criteria used to measure the same object (healthcare systems' performance in this case) is the result of a rather broad range of choices and invites us to think about how much less agreement there is about "what seems important" to us than we might expect. The same object can be viewed from different perspectives, believed (possibly) in good faith to be the best by each of their proponents even if they are not necessarily consistent with each other.

Hopes for information that can describe the complexity of a word in transformation have a lengthy history and intensified between the end of the nineteenth century and the beginning of the twentieth century with the appearance of new measurement tools, new statistical methods (Desrosières, 1998; Porter, 2003) and sampling strategies. In the subsequent years, technical advances have combined with shifting political balances to produce changes in how policies intended to assist the population are conceived and in public decision-making processes. The neoconservative thrust of the mid-1980s—incarnated symbolically by Margaret Thatcher in Europe and Ronald Reagan in the United States—had a sizable impact in the area of social security and welfare, ushering in a season of drastic cuts and a push to privatize the public assistance programs put in place after the Second World War. In parallel, new models for managing the public administration and healthcare, as in the case of New Public Management (NPM), put ever-greater emphasis on governing by numbers and on efficiency, while keeping the sharpest of eyes on mechanisms for curbing planned expenditure through complex outcome monitoring systems (Busso, 2015; Porter, 2003; Noto et al., 2020; Supiot, 2015). In an atmosphere of tension and turmoil, numbers seem to offer the agility needed to picture the state of the world with tools that support decisions by providing (apparently) neutral documentation of the possible outcomes, thus making it in fact possible to guide and monitor the activities of the various institutions. As we will see in the following pages, however, the concept of evaluation and how it is put into practice through indexes and indicators are very far from having the neutrality they claim, and often entail: "an intensely disciplining effect . . . generating outputs associated with the categories of efficiency and of optimizing the use of resources (the inputs), but at the same time almost entirely uninterested in identifying the more general outcomes of the action that has been taken on individuals' and institutions' lives" (Borghi & Giullari, 2015, p. 383).

If we are to gain any measure of understanding whatsoever of the unstoppable success of systems for measuring and classifying reality, the increasing use of rating systems, and the reliance on synthetic measures even when the data are variable or show limited reliability, we must take a broader view and abandon the idea that these phenomena should (or can) mirror reality and are thus capable of conveying a clear and unequivocally true to life image (Esposito & Stark, 2019). Ambivalence is etched deep in the relationship that advances in science and technology have brought about in modern societies, where growing differences and the coexistence of a plurality of actors who pursue divergent goals starting from equally divergent interests, orientations and ideas of value contribute to a heightened uncertainty, making it unrealistic to imagine, much less achieve, any shared order. "The world, society, life and personal identity are called ever more into question", as Berger & Luckmann emphasize, and each of the multiple interpretations that result defines its own perspectives of possible action (1995, p. 40). The many different possible perspectives and the continual search for meaning where there is no longer a consensus lay us open to insecurity and can lead to disorientation. The very faculty of reason that goes hand in hand with modernity presents itself, as Foucault notes, "as both despotism and enlightenment" (1985, p. 470), capable of bringing about results that were once unthinkable and, at the same time, of producing new risks. The transformation of forms of knowledge is emblematic of this standpoint: forms that are less and less likely to enable each of the actors to have direct experience of them. Though this has undeniable advantages—for example, by permitting linkages between contexts that are physically far apart— the informational basis seems "ever more intensely subject to forms of abstraction, representing itself as being embodied in procedures, standards, certification models and online platforms, as well as—and above all—in numbers, indexes, quantitative targets, grades and scores" (Borghi & Giullari, 2015, p. 381).

The idea that it is possible to rely on objective knowledge and that the governance of a society can be based on procedures that are objective (or whose lack of impartiality tends, as we will see, to be forgotten) is a myth that is deeply rooted in our conceptions of society, science and the ties that bind them to each other, both in scientific contexts and as regards politics and the many courses of action that can be taken through policies (Porter, 1995, 2003). Attempting to counter subjectivity and imagining that knowledge can free itself from the influence of vested interests or willful distortion thanks to the use of some sort of automatic mechanism—through "the reduction of judgement to a calculation" (Porter, 2003, p. 242), for example—helps reinforce the idea that governing by numbers can be inclusive and reduce inequalities (Berman & Hirschman, 2018). This idea of the role of institutions emerges from the ideal model contemplated by the Weberian conception of bureaucracy (Weber, 1922), emblem of the process of rationalization that took place at the beginning of the last century, when the impersonal order at the basis of the dealings between institutions and the public promised that everyone would receive similar services, without favoritism on the part of those in power that could advance some at the expense of others. As Weber himself acknowledges, however, these processes of rationalization and bureaucratization of society are by no means linear but produce outcomes that are open-ended, often problematic and inevitably ambivalent. The myth of technical knowledge and the discussion regarding its contradictions continued throughout the last century and is still present in the current debate about the role institutions play in dealing with the public in the healthcare sector as well as in other spheres, setting up a continuing tension between the ethical aspects of healthcare and the increasingly technical–procedural tack taken by its organization.

2 The ambivalence of measurement processes

On the basis of what Porter (2012) calls "the first law of funny numbers", all the successes of the processes that rely on quantitative data to describe reality are met with challenges to their reliability and charges that they may have been used instrumentally. Numbers are "funny"—as Porter tells us—because they are protean, not necessarily as objective and impartial as they often seem: indeed, they can become "dishonest" and contribute to altering the relationships of power between actors, not just as a result of intentional strategies. Each of the dimensions identified in the literature on ratings seems—as Esposito & Stark, for instance, argue—inevitably ambiguous, unsatisfactory and indispensable at one and the same time, and this leads to the apparent paradox that "the features for which ratings and rankings are rightly criticized are the same mechanisms that underlie their effectiveness" (Esposito & Stark, 2019, p. 5).

Nevertheless, aspects such as the hypersimplified representation of reality that data encourage or the inaccuracies in collecting and using information, not to mention the subjectivity of the criteria used in rankings—which are acknowledged to be unsatisfactory even by their authors—cannot be considered intrinsically negative, and their connotations vary according to the observer's point of view and the circumstances surrounding their use. Although assigning a score to the objects or organizations being assessed provides information based on a common metric which can be more readily circulated, this entails an inevitable loss of the information's distinctive, qualitative nuances. The negative connotation, however, is not the end of the story, and there is no lack of antecedents, as Esposito & Stark remind us, that demonstrate that using common, impersonal metrics may be relevant and useful. A case in point is that of money, which Simmel notes is an artifact capable of "expressing the value of each object with a number (its price) and making it comparable with every other object, regardless of its quality, its emotional value, and its position on the market" (Esposito & Stark, 2019, pp. 15–16).

Even the lack of transparency of which these systems are often accused has another side to it. It is usually regarded as negative, given that it is at odds with one of the most pervasive rhetoric about the shape that the relationship between institutions and the public ought to take because it can mask the processes used to select what defines the quality of a system, tilt the balance of power between the participants or conceal conflicts of interest between the evaluators and the evaluated (Esposito & Stark, 2019, p. 8; Dirindin et al., 2018). Not clarifying the dimensions that make up the final score, however, can also take on the opposite meaning if it makes it possible to prevent manipulation by the evaluated party (for instance, by preventing whoever produces the data from finessing them to match what they know will be judged positively) or to protect providers of confidential information. In this connection, Cooley and Snyder (2015) mention the case of the 2014 Corruption Perceptions Index,[2] which, in addition to drawing on official data and data produced by governments, also makes use of information from independent sources. Obviously, the latter have a central role, as no country wants to provide statistics documenting its corruption. In 2014, China dropped from 80th to 100th place on the index, enraging the country's government which, complaining that the index was not transparent, called its objectiveness and impartiality into question. Clearly, however, this lack of transparency had served to protect the sources of information from reprisals, which are not infrequent where corruption is endemic.

Despite the risks we have outlined, there is no escaping the need to define an appropriate space for representing phenomena where we believe action should be taken. As we will see shortly, even the act of description—which might be thought to be less problematic—is not free from complications.

2.1 *Good descriptions or descriptions of what's good?*

For a better understanding of these complications, a few words are in order regarding the far from straightforward nature of the activities involved in description. It is not just the reliance on numbers that muddies the picture: more generally, a role is also played by our expectation—often groundless—that what we intend to represent cannot help but correspond to the phenomenon that is its object. Description in any case means making a choice; it is not produced automatically but necessarily entails selecting the elements to be considered according to the goals we intend to pursue. Consequently, we cannot determine beforehand how much the information available to us will enable us to produce a good description, given that this outcome changes on the basis of the relational environment in which it takes shape, just as the availability of good information might not lead automatically to a description that matches its object. For example, descriptions may be false but still be accepted as positive. The relationship between the truth—a claimed objective correspondence with facts that are considered equally objective—and how good the description is thus cannot be taken for granted. An example can help clarify this. A distinction must be made, Sen argues, "between a description of something being good in the sense of being a good one *to give* and it being a good description of *that* thing" (1982, p. 434). To explain how this can be, Sen describes a paradoxical situation:

> The aspiring murderer demands from you a description of where his would-be victim has gone, and as you point at the wrong road he proceeds in that direction with a roar. That description of where the would-be victim has gone is, I would agree, a good one to give, but it can hardly be accepted as a good description of where the would-be victim has gone.
>
> (Sen, 1982, p. 434)

In the case of the murderer, it is easy to decide what side to take in providing information that is ethically correct, even if it is otherwise wrong. But deciding whether describing the situation in a way that does not correspond to the information at hand can be seen as equally legitimate in other circumstances is more complicated. If during the Covid-19 pandemic, the institutions had decided to give a description that soft-pedaled the situation so as not to alarm the public, would we consider it a "good description"? And would our opinion change if the motivations were economic, e.g., to be able to reopen businesses such as stores, restaurants and museums early so as to keep unemployment from spiking or prevent the tourism industry from collapsing? Whatever answer each of us thinks is most appropriate, the point is that a description (and how we judge it) depends on a composite set of circumstances, inextricably linked to the environment, the preferences, the goals and the values of the actors involved. And this invites us to think about the characteristics of the actors and the nature of their relationships (which we will mention only briefly here, to draw attention to the complications that must be borne in mind): for example, we should ask whether we can consider legitimate a paternalistic relationship between the institutions and the public in which the former can decide that it is best to keep the latter in the dark concerning how serious the situation really is in order to prevent widespread panic.

We could continue with many more examples, but the point is that the strategic games that using numbers permits are not always easy to reconstruct nor necessarily legitimate or acceptable to all. Reliance on "approximations, metaphors, simplifications, etc." can serve purposes that are just as relevant as empirically grounded arguments and, to determine how good the description is, we must pay attention to the specific circumstances surrounding it. In addition, organizations are complex environments, internally heterogeneous and freighted with strategic interaction where:

> Actors treat information opportunistically to pursue their own ends, which do not necessarily match those that they have stated. Withholding and concealing information, systematic distortion, dissimulation, sabotage and misrepresentation are all "information games" that the actors engaged in a planning process play recurrently and systematically. Not only are representing a problem and finding a solution not immune to these information handling strategies, but they often take place by these very means.
>
> (Lanzara, 1993, pp. 120–121)

Returning to numbers, while information is frequently subject to more or less intentional and/or acceptable misunderstandings and distortions, rankings and classification systems may also not aim primarily at describing reality. Indeed, they may serve other functions at the same time, such as that of establishing links and forms of dependence from what others who are considered significant are observing:

> The problem that ratings deal with is not observation of an independent world (for which they are inevitably flawed and inadequate) but the circularity of second-order observation in which observations must take into account the observations of others.
>
> (Esposito & Stark, 2019, p. 5)

The importance of the effects that these tools can produce does not depend so much on the expectation of having precise descriptions of the world as on the awareness that they are looked at by other people who operate in the same environment and whose judgments may be relevant. The centrality of this aspect also emerges from the multidisciplinary review of the literature on rankings we cited earlier, where the "comparative orderings perspective" that emphasizes how rankings stratify organizations and the individuals associated with them in terms of status and reputation occupies a key position (Rindova et al., 2018, p. 2176). In this case, there is a risk that description and evaluation—two different dimensions that should be kept separate—will overlap: it may be that even if an ordering is not the same as an evaluation, these two levels tend in actuality to coincide, and the position achieved in the ranking tends to be considered as an indicator of efficiency. For example, several studies have shown that students who graduate from universities regarded as prestigious—on the basis of their place in the rankings—have better career options regardless of whether they have in fact received a better education (Navarro, 2008; Rubin & Dierdorff, 2009, in Rindova et al., 2018), and that highly ranked businesses are able—with all other factors remaining equal—to increase their survival rates even during market crises (Rao, 1994; Sánchez et al., 2012; Rindova et al., 2018).

Though these aspects have been extensively documented in the literature, in practice the awareness of the distance separating objective description and representation frequently tends to evaporate, giving way to a sort of naturalization that makes representation take solid shape, and the cast shadows are mistaken for reality. Even if the actors know that the information is second-rate and whether it is well-founded cannot always be determined, and even if they are aware of the information's limits (inasmuch as it is often dated, incomplete or refers to periods that cannot be compared), the information nevertheless tends to acquire a weight that can impact the areas it claims to describe. In this interplay of reflected images that the actors cannot escape for fear of jeopardizing their reputations, the fact of being observed leads to what Espeland & Sauder call the reactivity of social measures: "the idea that people change their behavior in reaction to being evaluated, observed, measured" (2007, p. 1). In their analysis of the different components of reactivity, self-fulfilling prophecy[3] takes pride of place. Here, the effects that can be produced concern the possibility that even if rankings create hierarchies whose nature is difficult to determine and may be debatable, "They create lines that then have the danger of becoming real" (Espeland & Sauder, 2007, p. 12). Once produced, they can then engender a sort of lasting halo effect whereby "prior rankings shape current evaluation". More than how an organization functions today, it would thus be the score achieved in the past that determines how current performance is judged. Out of inertia, in cases where rankings are used as the basis for allocating resources, the same organizations will always receive more. Rewards based on the "best to best[4]" principle not only raise doubts about whether evaluation based more on the representation than on the substance makes sense but could also limit access to resources on the part of those who are most in need of them, thus preventing all of the organizations involved from being in a condition to at least attain a minimum acceptable standard.

3 The risks of measurement: gaming strategies

As we have said, relying on numbers is by no means the only way to make strategic use of information. Nevertheless, numbers seemingly convey a particularly robust and objective vision of reality. This is not a recent development. Many of the ambiguities and instrumental uses that still mark the reliance on numbers today can be traced to the early days of quantification processes. Porter (2012) reconstructs the use of statistics in dealing with mental patients since the 1830s and relates how Theodric Romeyn Beck collected data and published the first statistical reports showing that cure rates in America were comparable to those of the best-known European asylums of the time, causing conspicuous satisfaction among American asylum directors for the superiority of the outcomes of their treatment (Beck, 1830, in Porter, 2012, p. 588). The statistics about cures and patient characteristics were intended to make families understand how important it was to seek help from asylums for their relatives showing signs of mental illness before it was too late. Having figures that demonstrated asylums' effectiveness thus became particularly valuable, and the importance of the goals (curing early and better) seemed to justify pushing the figures' limits a bit, at least in the eyes of those who were doing the pushing. The numbers were thus frequently called on to provide the representation that was best suited to showing the asylum's success, in some cases even claiming that cure rates exceeded an already unrealistic 90%. With "funny numbers", the boundary between the patients' benefit and the fame of the institutions that accepted them was cleverly shifted. Even at the time, the high public visibility of numbers and statistics sparked heated discussions about their reliability and the legitimacy of their use: for example, Porter tells us that the German physician Maximilian Jacobi of the Siegburg Asylum believed that the implausibly high cure rates indicated by the English asylums' data had been artfully achieved by discharging patients before they had recovered (Pritchard, 1835, in Porter, 2012, p. 589). Porter also notes that the abrupt drop in "cures" in Massachusetts occasioned vigorous complaints by asylum officials, who maintained that they had been forced to take patients in such serious condition that there was no hope of helping them. So as not to see their reputations jeopardized, the asylums worked their magic with the numbers, manipulating them in a "statistical alchemy, transforming a death into a discharge". Reclassification thus made it possible for the asylums to even deny death, hiding it among the discharges or carefully avoiding to account for the percentage of relapsed patients and artificially upping their cure rates (Porter, 2012, pp. 589–590).

Porter does not deny the importance of using numbers to compare different organizations' performance. However, in demonstrating the ambiguities that this involves, he invites us to gain a better understanding of the outcomes, for example by casting light on the relational effects accompanying them and the historically situated nature of whatever phenomena are being analyzed. The " 'dark side' of rankings as instruments of surveillance and control" (Rindova et al., 2018) has effects we should be aware of. A very high cure rate or a good position in the rankings can come about for many different reasons. Though these reasons obviously include good treatment and exceptional performance, we cannot rule out other circumstances such as the fact that organizations can learn to adapt their own performance to what the ranking systems regard as right, producing an entire chain of consequences. Thus, the organizations' own purposes may be shunted into the background, and chasing after "improved rankings as an explicit goal" (Espeland & Sauder, 2007, p. 15) takes priority. The point is that the very fact of having an evaluation system changes the outlook of the people and organizations involved. For example, in their case study of law school rankings, Espeland and Sauder found that introducing two indicators of placement at and after graduation resulted in more time being invested in tracking student employment, time that was inevitably taken from other activities:

> While students clearly benefit from career services departments that are extremely motivated to help them find jobs, there are drawbacks to this emphasis on statistics. Personnel complain that time spent on tracking students' job status decreases time spent counseling students, networking with law firms, and conducting employment seminars. One director estimated she spent one day every week on employment statistics.
>
> (Espeland & Sauder, 2007, p. 27)

The fact that organizations participating in ranking systems are incentivized "to focus their efforts on improving their relative position rather than investing in their own strategic visions" (Rindova et al., 2018, p. 2177) produces substantial changes within the organization. These changes, however, take place almost through inertia and in response to seemingly neutral requests. On the other hand, the stakes are so high that they also make it more likely that the actors will resort to gaming, a strategy that "is about managing appearances and involves efforts to improve ranking factors without improving the characteristics the factors are designed to measure" (Espeland & Sauder, 2007, p. 129). Such strategies are particularly significant, not only because they widen the gap between the evaluation and the organization's real characteristics but also because they are considered illegitimate and thus encourage concealment and secrecy (since what is going on cannot be made public) and also contribute to eroding the relations between organizations subject to the same ranking system, as they breed distrust about what the others might be doing (Bevan & Hood, 2006).

All of this leads to consequences that raise rather weighty ethical questions. Is it legitimate to change the representation of reality to achieve results that a certain community considers important? And if it is, under what circumstances? Who do we think should be given the power to decide? Whatever answers may be possible, it should be emphasized that they must necessarily hinge on the characteristics of the specific contexts where these questions arise.

4 A sector to be sheltered

The sectors of public importance—like healthcare—belong to what the Foundational Economy[5] considers areas "to be sheltered", and where "we would expect—or rather, we should expect—that the ends pursued by economic actors adhere strictly to the idea of *social utility*" (Barbera et al., 2016, p. 67). Leaving aside for the moment the heterogeneity underlying the concept of social utility (to which we will return in Chapter 3), it is precisely in sectors of this kind that uncontrolled gaming can produce especially jarring outcomes, at times explicitly driven by an ideological hyper-efficiency where cutting costs trumps looking after the public's wellbeing. In the following examples, we will illustrate the risks in contexts—the United States, Italy and the United Kingdom—which, though they have very different healthcare models, demonstrate how pervasive these risks are. The examples also show how the outcomes they produce do not depend so much on the specific characteristics of the individuals involved as on normative and cultural environments that can impel certain lines of conduct rather than others.

We will start from the United States. Here, in 2004, 186 interventional cardiologists included in the 1998–2000 Percutaneous Coronary Interventions report, a disclosure of physician-specific performance data that New York State has published since 1994, were asked to complete a short questionnaire to assess whether having the outcomes of their work (including patient mortality rates following coronary angioplasty) made public had had any effect on their clinical practice.[6] Of the 120 cardiologists who agreed to participate in the survey, 79% admitted that their decision on whether to perform angioplasty on critically ill patients could be influenced by the knowledge that the outcomes of surgery are shown on their physician scorecards (Narins et al., 2005).

The second example, which passed somewhat under the radar in Italy, concerns a decision of the president of the Istituto Nazionale della Previdenza Sociale (INPS), the Italian social security administration (INPS, *2018–2020 Performance Plan*, decision No. 24 of March 13, 2018) which sets out the targets that physicians are required to reach in order to qualify for certain types of supplemental pay. One of the conditions for receiving incentives was revoking disability allowances, a set of benefits that includes a monthly payment to individuals affected by congenital or acquired conditions that limit their ability to work. For taking these benefits away from patients, physicians were thus rewarded with a sum that could be quite sizable.[7] By contrast, the disability specialists on the medical boards that assess patients' condition receive much less, approximately 50 euros gross per board session (generally lasting four to five hours), or around ten euros gross per hour, corresponding to a net hourly rate of seven euros. On the basis of the plan's content, it would thus appear that those who decide whether to grant benefits to the disabled are rewarded if they do not do so, while those who could safeguard the rights in question are in practice discouraged from doing their part. Though no data is available concerning the action actually taken by physicians and there are no compelling reasons to believe that individuals act in expectation of higher pay alone (Frey, 1997), the context points to misaligned incentives that provide economic advantages which run counter to professional ethics. As the physician who drew attention to the case wrote:

> It is not difficult to image what the consequences of the guidelines laid out in the president's decision might be: when the medical board physicians employed or associated with INPS are called upon to assess an individual's level of disability, their own private economic interests will clash with their professional duty to act according to science and conscience.
>
> (Agnoletto, 2018)

The third example comes from a paper tellingly entitled "What's measured is what matters", in which Bevan & Hood document the increase in gaming during the years when Britain's National Health Service gradually morphed into a target system where:

> Desired results are specified in advance in measurable form, some system of monitoring measures performance against that specification, and feedback mechanisms are linked to measured performance.
>
> (2006, p. 5)

The system uses various kinds of rewards and sanctions, including:

> reputational effects (shame or glory accruing to managers on the basis of their reported performance); bonuses and renewed tenure for managers that depend on performance against target; "best to best" budgetary allocations that reflect measured performance; and the granting of "earned autonomy" (from detailed inspection and oversight) to high performers.
>
> (Bevan & Hood, 2006, p. 6)

The authors provide many well-documented examples of the changes the system has brought about; however, although they point out that the majority of managers and physicians show little inclination to take advantage of the opportunities the system offers them, and the percentage of documented instances of gaming is small, they also stress that the organization exerts a pressure such "that governance by targets can turn 'knights' into 'knaves' by rewarding those who produce the right numbers for target achievement" (LeGrand, 2003, in Bevan & Hood, 2006, p. 9). For example, introducing a performance indicator requiring that 75% of ambulances must reach patients within eight minutes (in the case of Category A calls for immediately life-threatening emergencies) resulted in a significant increase in response times meeting this target, but no substantial improvement in waiting times, or even in patient care:

> A study by the Commission for Health Improvement (2003) found evidence that in a third of ambulance trusts, response times had been "corrected" to be reported to be less than eight minutes. . . . There was also evidence that the idiosyncrasies of the rules about Category A classification led in some instances to patients in urgent need being given a lower priority for ambulance response than less serious cases that happened to be graded Category A.
>
> (Bevan & Hood, 2006, p. 19)

The cases we have presented illustrate concrete risks for the wellbeing of patients, whose condition should be aided rather than used to reach other types of goal. They also show that the instrumental use of data can become "normal"—as a result of superficiality or as an automatic reaction—and that consequently it is not sufficiently called out or monitored. Habits encourage processes of naturalization that reduce the range of possibilities, clearing the way for an interpretation of what is going on that is less likely to be questioned. This is the issue we will discuss in the following section.

5 Regarding the naturalization of the way we observe reality

The alchemy worked by rankings and measurement systems is not limited to bringing about changes in behavior in response to something that is considered to be real, as in the case of self-fulfilling prophesies. Something additional is also produced in more subtle ways, by altering—through commensuration—the cognitive mechanisms whereby we assign importance to certain factors and deny it to others: "Commensuration is characterized by the transformation of qualities into quantities . . . shapes what we pay attention to, which things are connected to other things, and how we express sameness and difference" (Espeland & Sauder, 2007, p. 16). When information is simplified and decontextualized, much of its content tends to seem irrelevant and what remains becomes more authoritative, to the point that it appears inevitable and self-evident. Through commensuration and simplification, a complex concept such as the quality of an organization is condensed into a number that appears "more robust and definitive than it would if presented in more complicated forms" (Espeland & Sauder, 2007, p. 17). Espeland & Sauder note that several decades earlier, Simmel (1971) had observed that, as a result of the processes that lead us to consider a certain social form as natural, any other alternative tends to seem unreal. The anxiousness to measure, as well as the ambivalence of measurements, contributes to creating an environment where, to cope with the resulting uncertainty "our minds play all sorts of tricks on us, and we on them[8]" (Elster, 1983, p. 111). After we have made a choice, for example, our preferences may change to avoid regretting the option we did not choose, thus reinforcing the polarization between opposites, as a way of reducing cognitive dissonance (Festinger, 1957). This process produces an evaluation that accentuates the presumed negative attributes of the rejected option, though this is not necessarily an intentional outcome or one of which the participants are conscious:

> Every preference for a possible order is accompanied, most often implicitly, by the aversion for the opposite possible order. That which diverges from the preferable in a given area of evaluation is not the indifferent but the repulsive or more exactly, the repulsed, the detestable. . . . In short, norms, whether in some implicit or explicit form, refer the real to values, express discrimination of qualities in conformity with the polar opposition of a positive and a negative.
>
> (Canguilhem, 1978, p. 147)

In this connection, Foucault speaks of "a ritual of manifestation of the truth" which goes beyond a "more or less rational activity of knowledge"; what is involved is a set of procedures "by which one brings to light . . . something that is asserted or rather laid down as true" (2014, p. 6). What takes shape in each instance is what Maurizio Ferraris calls an interpretive scheme, viz.:

> the action taken in the world and on the world (natural and social) without concepts but not without effects, through a competence without understanding which characterizes much of our being in the world far more often than does having concepts.
>
> (2017, p. 142)

Events and our understanding of what happens are "captured" by the interpretive scheme and thus by the perspective or the role of whoever is doing the choosing, selecting some of the various possible perspectives. Through commensuration, rankings simultaneously *unify*—given that they iron out differences by establishing a common metric—and *distinguish*, through the position organizations occupy in the hierarchy that the ranking sets up. The resulting image of the world is "taken as true", it does not seem to create problems nor trigger reactions; it assumes a normative and prescriptive dimension that is no longer questioned, becoming natural and appearing normal. The processes of normalization that take place as society's functioning is shaped and controlled (Foucault, 1999) are complex, because in addition to helping produce a common meaning that makes a certain course of action and the way things are both obvious and taken for granted, it brings about a sort of *"cognitive hegemony*, so spectacularly characterized by the *power to otherize* anything that deviates from a certain standard", without this being seen as problematic (Zerubavel, 2018, p. 58) or without its bias being perceived.

The naturalization of the meanings that circulate in society can thus depend on many reasons that are at least to some extent unconnected with the intentions of the actors involved. We look at the classifications that recommend a certain restaurant not so much because it does not occur to us that they might be fake, but because we are in a hurry or because as far as we know they might even be true; or again, because—in some way that we do not entirely understand—they help keep our uncertainty about the choice within bounds. In this case, though, the stakes are rather low, and if the restaurant turns out to be bad we can always pan it in a review of our own or decide never to set foot there again.

Other areas—as we mentioned earlier—pose different problems. In the field of public policy, taking for granted a certain interpretation and a certain course of action, or a certain quantity of resources that is considered good inasmuch as it is less than some previous amount means assuming that alternatives are not feasible and, in practice, espousing the idea that there are in fact no possible alternatives. As is clear from what is happening to our collective ability to face the Covid-19 pandemic that is now wreaking havoc, the fact that we have spent the last several decades taking for granted that there is no alternative to drastic cuts to welfare systems, assuming that privatizing the healthcare system, shedding personnel and reducing the number of hospital beds were the only possible answers and accepting that all this was inevitable has done a disservice to our capacity for agency in a field as crucial as public health. Having reduced "the possible in the real" (Borghi, 2019) seems to have contributed to producing the painful consequences that are now afflicting us. As Borghi reminds us, we can and must start by studying the complex relationship between experience, knowledge and information in order to understand the role that infrastructures of experience (such as ranking systems, but more generally all mechanisms that assume a sort of mechanical and unquestioned objectivity while also claiming to be rigorously neutral) play in predetermining the meanings assigned to what we consider valuable. Recovering room for agency means remembering that the cognitive domain of institutions (De Leonardis, 2001), pervasive though it may be, is not inescapable:

> the infrastructures through which we experience are something in which we are thrown, a sort of "second nature"; but they are also the product of human activity, the result of the work of individuals who, with different responsibilities, perform tasks, develop projects, use techniques and technologies. This perspective opens the black box of expertise, of the transformation of normative issues in techno-bureaucratic matter and exposes to critical scrutiny the evaluation criteria embodied in the apparently neutral devices and routines our activities are based on.
>
> (Borghi, 2019, p. 43)

Institutions wield what Pizzorno calls "the terrible power of identifying" (2007) terrible because it is omnipresent and able to produce major consequences, for example, in establishing what is legitimate and what is not, what is normal and what is not. The actors nevertheless still have some margin for agency, though variable according to circumstances. Observing and trying to understand what goes on in the black box of normalization processes and in the dynamics—more or less binding—that link institutions and the public thus calls for reconstructing the actors' interests and motivations and the far from predictable outcomes that their concrete form can produce (Bosco, 2006). In the case of rankings, this involves paying attention to how they build up a reference audience (Esposito & Stark, 2019) or, as Rindova and colleagues suggest (2018), training our gaze on ranking entrepreneurship, or in other words on the characteristics and the activities of the collective actors that initiate and develop ranking systems. In the case of healthcare (but not only there), focusing on those who have the power to influence the choice of indicators makes it possible to observe the complex equilibriums that take place in healthcare systems between actors pursuing potentially conflicting interests. As a result of the power to define that producers of rankings enjoy and the cognitive hegemony they are able to establish (Zerubavel, 2018), major international institutions could, for example, underestimate the impact on quality that can be exerted by the more specific and local goals of different national systems as regards the public's needs. Concentrating on the complex nature of the actors and the interests pursued by each can help in piecing together a better understanding of opaque processes and the gulf separating them from the straightforward, consensus-based and rational image that we fondly believe (or would like) information to have.

6 Gaming strategies and conflicts of interest in healthcare

The many different interests at play in healthcare make for a particularly delicate relationship between the parties who are entitled to determine where choices must be made and the arguments that will be used to justify them to the public. Naturally, this plurality of interests widens the array of objectives that can be pursued, inevitably complicating a picture featuring such dissimilar stakeholders: the multinational pharmaceutical companies seeking to maximize profits, the public healthcare system's political actors and administrators who are concerned with overall financial sustainability, frontline healthcare personnel who would like to be guaranteed better working conditions and the most modern technologies and the patients who concentrate on improving their condition. And the equilibria between these actors are constantly shifting. Though they obviously depend on the power held by each actor, they can also be changed further as a result of outside causes. The current pandemic, for example, seems to have created an unusual and perhaps unprecedented alliance of interests in defense of the public system (at least in the public discourse). In addition, a number of hoary arguments have been called into question, such as the putative superiority of an efficient private sector over an inefficient public system or the "need" for cuts. It is still too early to know whether this is a substantive change that will result in greater attention to the public functions of healthcare systems and the central importance of safeguarding them. There is no lack of worrisome signals of corruption and organized crime infiltration in healthcare contracts or of frauds exploiting a fearful public.[9]

The circumstances call for caution, and it is perhaps worth recalling the remarks made in 2016 by Raffaele Cantone, then president of Italy's National Anti-Corruption Authority. At an event marking the first National Day Against Corruption in Healthcare, Cantone noted that "healthcare is a hunting ground for criminals of all kinds, a world of enormous economic interests even in times of crisis" (Gobbi, 2016). According to the OECD (2017), corruption and conflicts of interest are widespread problems in many countries that can divert a significant proportion of healthcare expenditures.[10]

In healthcare relationships, conflicts of interest[11] can produce a shift away from what is widely seen as the primary interest—"reaching the best possible state of health for the patient"—toward secondary interests. The latter can include "the widest variety of economic and financial returns, personal interests, political objectives and religious conventions that can influence healthcare workers' judgement in reaching the interest that should guide their decisions" (Dirindin et al., 2018, p. 23). Though the distinction between primary and secondary interests is not the same as that between conditions that can be considered acceptable and those that cannot—given that the actors involved have a range of other legitimate interests—the power advantage that some parties enjoy can have important consequences for patients. Given the inconstant equilibrium between primary and secondary interests and the possibility that they can come into conflict, it is quite likely that whichever is stronger will prevail. Information has a central role in this dynamic. Information gaps, as Dirindin and colleagues (2018) point out, are ingrained in healthcare, where information is not only difficult to reconstruct but also changes constantly. Even research is part of an unending process whose coordinates cannot be fully mastered even by the experts. Nevertheless, these gaps can create major risks in terms of both efficiency and fairness:

> those who have more information naturally tend to use it for their own advantage, and not only to benefit others who turn to them because of their greater knowledge, producing suboptimal effects and reducing the protection afforded to the weakest.
>
> (Dirindin et al., 2018, p. 22)

Information asymmetry is at the roots of many aspects of corruption and medical malpractice, and the risks can increase if there is no widespread awareness of the weight that unequal access to information can have in influencing health outcomes. In 2017, a survey entitled "Curiamo la corruzione" (We Treat Corruption) by Transparency International Italy, Censis, ISPE Sanità and RiSSC found that—despite the evidence for corruption—it is not widely perceived as a problem by the officers in charge of preventing corruption in healthcare facilities: 64.7% of the interviewees stated that the risk of corruption at their own unit was moderate, while only 5.9% felt that there was a high risk (Report Curiamo la corruzione, 2017). In addition to being an ethical problem, corruption entails a significant cost for the healthcare system and drains further resources from a long-beleaguered sector. It also has major consequences on how conflicts of interest play out, as it makes it more likely that the strongest will gain the upper hand. Confirming how vital an awareness of information is, it should be emphasized that conflicts of interest often hinge on information and the ways in which its coordinates and circulation can be controlled. Skewed information can cause conflicts of interest to arise in a broad range of circumstances: in clinical practice, for example, when drug salesmen incentivize physicians to prescribe particular medications or treatments; in scientific research and its dissemination (Bobbio, 2004, 2017); in the activities of scientific societies or patients' associations; in the administration of tender competitions and contracts (Dirindin et al., 2018, pp. 28–29). In the pharmaceutical market, health systems are increasingly unable to exercise control over private economic interests in such matters as setting drug prices (Canduro, 2018). As Dirindin and colleagues emphasize in this connection, "The literature offers extensive evidence of the link between pharmaceutical marketing and the overdiagnosis of conditions that, if no drug existed, would not be considered health problems" (2018, p. 56). Artificial needs can thus be created through marketing campaigns that not only invent the need but also show how it can be resolved. As for the actual needs—for access to new drugs, for example—international pharmaceutical companies can succeed in charging exorbitant prices by concealing the real production costs and fielding complex negotiation strategies with individual countries without revealing the terms agreed upon in others. The novel antiviral sofosbuvir used to treat hepatitis C with very high viral suppression rates is one example out of many: in 2014, a 12-week course of the drug cost $84,000 in the United States. Production costs at that time, however, were 99.8% below the price charged on the market, which would have permitted the same course of treatment to be provided for less than $200 (Hill et al., 2016).

While vested interests are to some extent inevitable, Big Pharma's power outweighs that of the organisms—both national and international—that should monitor the industry's doings and put mechanisms in place for controlling them. In some cases, the presence of actors with potentially conflicting interests is legitimated and normalized, as when industry sponsorship of medical societies' conferences is disclosed on the societies' websites (Fabbri et al., 2016), while in other cases it can take stealthier forms—whose effectiveness is directly proportionate to how hidden they are—that can even influence the areas chosen for research and dictate its outcomes:

> the evidence based "quality mark" has been misappropriated and distorted by vested interests. In particular, the drug and medical devices industries increasingly set the research agenda. They define what counts as disease . . . and predisease "risk states" . . . . They also decide which tests and treatments will be compared in empirical studies and choose (often surrogate) outcome measures for establishing "efficacy".
>
> (Greenhalgh et al., 2014)

For new drugs—whose efficacy should be determined through research—the centers that carry out clinical trials may thus be asked to conduct equivalence trials to "determine, not that a new therapy is 'superior', but that it is 'not inferior' to current standard therapies" (Dirindin et al., 2018, p. 57). This practice—widely regarded as unethical—makes it possible to market products that are "not much worse than the available standard products", but are essentially useless and create an artificial need for themselves (Garattini & Bertelé, 2007, in Dirindin et al., 2018).

Lastly, no discussion of potential conflicts of interest and how information affects their outcomes should fail to mention the role of private insurance companies, who find fertile ground in the narratives that play up the unsustainability of public health services, presenting their failures and cases of malpractice as representative of their operation in general and taking for granted that private is always better than public (Carraro & Quezel, 2018). Opportunistically emphasizing public healthcare's shortcomings, however, is dangerous, as it tends to further naturalize the absence of alternatives, clearing the way for massive profits from private health insurance coverage.

As we have seen in the foregoing pages, the role of information in healthcare (and in all areas of importance to the community as a whole) is crucial and calls for a closer look. We will scrutinize this role, and the relationship between information and public decisions, in the following pages. But first, a short summary of what we have seen so far may be useful.

Our lengthy digression on systems for classifying and describing the reality that surrounds us was intended to draw attention to the ambivalent nature of reality and the—equally ambivalent—nature of the information we have for describing it. Though the Italian National Health Service's uneven scores in the ranking systems might have us believe otherwise, it is not the best of its ilk and neither is it the worst. It is important to bear in mind, however, that it is still a universalist system, despite years of cuts and retrenchments that have narrowed its scope and called its basic assumptions into question. It is fraught with complex and inevitably ambivalent relationships that can result in processes of exclusion and heighten inequalities. It has been put under pressure by actors who pursue legitimate secondary interests, but much less legitimately give these interests priority over the primary need to safeguard the health of patients and the public. Consequently, it is in need of protection and shelter, and information is a major resource for monitoring its characteristics and outcomes. It is by being alert to information that we can gain the knowledge needed, case by case, to preserve the system. But we tend to forget that information itself is riddled with ambiguities.

Notwithstanding all evidence to the contrary, being able to rely on objective, believable reconstructions still seems necessary, useful and reassuring. To take an example: it is April 2020, the Covid-19 pandemic is in full swing, and every evening at 6:00 the Italian Civil Defense Department—the public agency coordinating and monitoring the efforts to curb the virus' spread—calls a press conference to present the latest news about the situation, with the number of new cases, recovered patients and deaths in the last 24 hours. We all wait for the daily bulletin on tenterhooks, even if it is not at all clear what these figures mean: given the shortage of swab tests, the number of new cases cannot in fact be calculated, since it reflects how much testing can be done every day; recovered patients may not really have recovered, since some experts believe that the virus can return and, at least in one region, it has been pointed out that they are counted together with the patients being cared for at home after discharge and who continue to be positive[12]; new deaths do not include cases where no swab test was done or where it was not possible to certify the cause of death, as well as the hundreds of elderly patients who died in care homes. According to some estimates (Ricolfi, 2020), if all these cases were counted the total number of deaths would be two, five, seven or ten times higher, depending on the area of the country. But even if we are aware of the ambiguities, it is not easy to shake off the fascination that numbers (and certain narratives) exert on us. Under what conditions, then, can we put our trust in information during public decision-making processes?

7 Does information help us decide[13]?

In "Development as Freedom", Sen tells a parable about a woman—Annapurna—who wants someone to clear up her garden, and must choose between three people who would do the job in much the same way and at much the same cost. The only problem is that the work cannot be distributed among the three, so she will have to choose only one. The woman, Sen tells us, thus asks herself who would be right to employ, given that all three are poor, and the job would be very important in improving conditions for any of them.

If the only thing Annapurna knew was that all of them are poor, she could choose at random, and the job could be given to any of the three. But she also knows something about their lives and that there are significant differences between them as regards the benefit they would derive from being able to work. Which of the candidates, then, on the basis of the information available to Annapurna, would it be right to hire? Dinu is the poorest of the three, and Annapurna asks herself: "What can be more important . . . than helping the poorest?" Bishanno is psychologically the most depressed: he has only recently been impoverished and has not yet been able to adjust to the fact. If he were to be given the job, he would be the one who stands to gain most in "happiness". Here again, there is a good reason to have him do the job, since Annapurna tells herself that "Surely removing unhappiness has to be . . . the first priority". The third prospect, Rogini, is debilitated from a chronic ailment, and if she got the job, she could use the money to rid herself of the disease. Though she is not as poor as the others, in her case the job "would make the biggest difference . . . to the quality of life and freedom from illness" (Sen, 1999, p. 55).

For Annapurna, as we have said, the problem is to make the "right" choice, which, from her point of view, means benefiting the one who is in the greatest need of the three, and also the one whose life would be most improved. With the story of Annapurna, Sen runs through the arguments in the theoretical debate about justice and anticipates many of the questions that public institutions must address when setting priorities for action. The need to decide between different alternatives when resources are scarce—in the parable, there is not enough work for everyone who needs it—is par for the course for institutions. But there is a further point that should be emphasized in thinking about the relationship between information and choice. If Annapurna had had less information, the choice would have been easy: if she had known, for example, only who was poorest, with all else being equal, she would have had no difficulty deciding. But she knows about everyone's condition, each of which would in itself have made it reasonable to give the job—or allocate the available resources, in other words—to the person in that condition.

It might seem that the detailed information that Annapurna has is a double-edged sword, as far as its consequences are concerned: the difficulty depends on having alternatives that are hard to order on a hierarchical scale. In a situation like this, then, it seems that information brings more problems than it solves. But is this really true? And what is the relationship between knowledge and choice?

In the light of Sen's tale, we could argue that Annapurna has taken a "responsible" approach to the problem facing her: she collects information, formulates questions and tries to find answers that are consistent with her goal of making a fair choice, starting from what she knows about the situation. If we imagine that instead of Annapurna we have a hospital that has to decide how to allocate public resources, the question becomes: what should a public choice that avoids taking sides and seeks the greatest good for the community be like? And what kind of justification for the choices can be considered responsible?

The implications of Sen's story are important on several levels. Gaining information is not a zero-cost process. Given that public choices must also be publicly justified, communicating them calls for particular caution, as regards both methods and content. But one thing at a time. The first problem has to do with the relationship between knowledge and decision.

As we saw, having a lot of information or, as we might say, having options that are not easy to order hierarchically, does not help Annapurna to decide. Quite frequently, in fact, we come up against *irreducible conflicts of compelling principles* (Sen, 1987), where it is impossible to arrive at a *balanced complete ordering of the alternatives*, or in other words decide whether "*on balance* one alternative combination of objects is superior to another" (Sen, 1987, p. 65). Here, several situations can arise: (a) the decision-maker may be unable to order preferences that involve—as in Annapurna's case—contradictory principles and different conceptions of utility and (b) it may be difficult to order contrasting principles when the choice must be agreed upon by several actors each of whom more or less consciously holds an idea contrasting with those of the others. However, we may also have situation (c) where it is hard to choose not so much because of the difficulty in ordering contrasting preferences or principles, but because it is necessary to establish which information—out of the mass of information available—is relevant in the light of principles that are considered to be clear.

Another factor that makes having information ambiguous is that it seems to increase the uncertainty about our choices' purposes (as in Annapurna's case) and about the effects of our actions. And this could make it "rational" to abandon our attempts at rationality. As Sen tells us: "If most of the important things that happen are not intended (and not brought about through purposive action), then reasoned attempts at pursuing what we want might appear to be rather pointless" (1999, p. 250).

It is thus no easy matter to accept our limits, nor to come to terms with the *Unsicherheit*[14] that weighs ever more heavily on our lives.[15] Against a backdrop of growing ambiguity and indeterminacy, the relationship between information and choice can unfold in two opposite ways: the first consists in declaring that information is irrelevant, whereas the second and converse approach assigns importance to the data collected in order to orient choices. And as we mentioned earlier, the need to publicly justify choices adds a further difficulty.

The first possibility thus means implementing strategies—which may or may not be done consciously—for removing, eliminating or shifting the risk and the associated insecurity. In the area of health and welfare policies—and the discourses surrounding them—this can entail giving up on collecting information and asking questions for which the only answers are incomplete and consequently unsatisfactory. This route, however, is likely to lead to commonsense discourses that are not supported by reasonably well-grounded evidence, like the indisputable need for cuts, the superior efficiency of the private sector, the system's unsustainability and so forth. This solution can be seen as *culturally relativistic*, inasmuch as it does not explicitly take a definite ethical stance (it does not argue, for example, that a given percentage of expenditure is better because it is "fair") but risks shading into a sort of "moral indifference" that suspends judgment even though it does not abstain from choosing (for instance, by claiming that a certain percentage of debt to GDP or across-the-board cuts in the number of hospital beds are unavoidable).

Not collecting information, however, is also compatible with a stance that is diametrically opposed to cultural relativism. This is a perspective that shares the idea that information is irrelevant with the relativist approach, but by contrast with the latter, presupposes the *universality of culture* and relies heavily on values which, if assumed to be universal, need no validation. Here again, it is not necessary to gather data and information, since the criteria are not established on the basis of the information we have but are implicit in the fact that these specific values are assumed:

> In assuming a precise standard of evaluation and judgement, policies are not "morally indifferent". As this standard remains largely implicit (or tends to become implicit over time), it has all the weight of the natural, the obvious, part of the way things are: the hierarchy implicit in these policies is naturalized, the ethical aspect of choosing the point of view is concealed in "the way things are".
>
> (Pitch, 2001)

Thus, although the basic assumptions are universalistic, once again the door may be left open to a proliferation of discursive milieux that are not only unsubstantiated, but are not believed to require substantiation. Examples include the absolute contrast between good and evil, between healthy and diseased, between worthy and unworthy, between those who see protecting the public's health as all-important and those whose major concern is getting the economy going again.

A second—and decidedly less common—way of looking at the relationship between information and choice involves accepting the risk that inevitably accompanies uncertainty. This leads to the attempt to identify feasible routes (chiefly public routes) that embrace—rather than reject—efforts to find new outlooks, new ways of thinking, of formulating questions and hazarding answers. To decide to invest in collecting information, it is necessary to recognize that these two approaches are alternatives and select the second, with all the inevitable "risks" it brings.

The problem is that in the case of public choices, the absolutely rational approach—collecting all the information and then deciding—is not immediately applicable, as it poses numerous problems. Indeed, we are dealing here with models of choice whose feasibility depends on particularly restrictive conditions that, as Luigi Bobbio points out, "rarely present themselves simultaneously in administrative life" (1996, p. 18). For example, it is assumed that the ends (in the current pandemic, should these ends be protecting the economy or safeguarding health?) can be determined before the means for reaching them are identified or that decisions can be based on relatively stable conditions that enable us to analyze the alternatives and their consequences. While it is true that the assumptions about applying synoptic rationality to decisions have been superseded by models based on procedural and bounded forms of rationality, it is nevertheless undeniable that "the idea of rational government is one of the greatest aspirations (or one of the most powerful myths) of Western political culture" (Bobbio, 1996, p. 15). Here we are navigating a terrain bounded on one side by an awareness of the limits of an approach that relies on synoptic rational choice models and on the other by the ever-present likelihood of a slide into relativism which would erode all hope of anchoring our choices to any kind of defensibly empirical foundation. The problem seems to be as follows: if knowledge does not automatically help us choose, how is it possible to anchor our choices to a mooring that is even remotely solid without making these choices from the perspective of absolute rationality and without falling into an absolute relativism that makes reliance on reason superfluous?

Though we have long since moved beyond the positivist conception of knowledge as a process of progressive sedimentation, built up layer after layer, which through the full control of nature makes it possible to plan and monitor the goals to be achieved, this perspective is still deeply rooted in our cognitive universe. On the one hand, we admit that "the progress of knowledge does nothing but bring greater uncertainty" (Adam, 1999, p. 53; Giddens, 1990); on the other, we frequently find ourselves wanting to remove this awareness from our cognitive horizon. There is thus an unresolved tension between being aware of the general inapplicability of approaches based on absolute rationality and actually shelving them once and for all. Indeed, rational choice theory is still "the main framework for the social sciences". In part, this is because rationality, in all its possible shapes, continues to be first and foremost a normative ideal:

> We would all like to be rational, and we are certainly not proud of our occasional lapses from rationality, in the form of illusions or weaknesses of the will. Secondly, rationality is the assumption behind every hermeneutic act. To understand others' behavior, we must assume that they are rational beings on the whole. Without this assumption, we would not be able to attribute the desires and convictions to them that we use as the basis for interpreting behavior.
>
> (Elster, 1997, p. 230)

But at this point, what route can we take that will enable us to make the most of the information we have and use it in a way that is both "cautious and careful"? Once again, Sen comes to our aid. After a rundown of the reasons for being skeptical about rationality, he reaches the conclusion that "the possibility of reasoned progress" (1999, p. 249) still exists. Here we will focus on only one[16] of the objections that Sen discusses and his counterarguments, viz., the contention that the unintended consequences of choices cannot be controlled. To dismantle this objection, Sen makes a distinction between *unintended consequences* and *unpredictable consequences*. The fact that consequences may be unintended—he maintains—can scarcely be surprising, since "Any action has very many consequences, and only some of them could have been intended by the actors" (Sen, 1999, p. 256).

And these consequences may be positive or negative. Consequences may be unintended, but this does not mean that they could not have been predicted:

> If this is the way the idea of unintended consequences is understood (in terms of *anticipation* of important but unintended consequences), it is no way hostile to the possibility of rationalist reform. In fact, quite the contrary. Economic and social reasoning can take note of consequences that may not be intended, but which nevertheless result from institutional arrangements, and the case for particular institutional arrangements can be better evaluated by noting the likelihood of various unintended consequences.
>
> (Sen, 1999, p. 257)

It is thus possible to take a medium-range approach to public decision-making that uses the tools of rational choice, assigns importance to information and communicating it, and is at the same time aware that it is not possible to have absolute control over the effects of the action that has been taken (and is perhaps not interested in exerting control even if it were possible). The rationality that Sen invites us to consider is procedural[17] and entails keeping an eye on the intermediate goals that have been achieved, which gives us feedback so we can "adjust our aim".[18] Recognizing that decisions can only be partial does not exempt us from paying attention to the consequences that can arise from our action, and realize "the importance of studying unintended effects. . ., and it would be a complete mistake to think that the importance of unintended effects undermines the need for rational assessment of all effects—unintended as well as intended" (Sen, 1999, pp. 260–261). According to Sen, then, information matters, as it is the only compass we have for trying to determine where we want to go and what route we will take to get there. Even if we are aware that the information we have collected falls short of what we need in order to decide, we thus cannot avoid using it and finding ways to justify what we are doing. Annapurna's attitude is responsible (but the same could be true for a collective actor), in that it does not eliminate the complexity but makes every effort to find the way that is subjectively best for coming to terms with it. Being responsible requires that we agree at least on the fact that it is necessary to have pertinent information before making a choice. Once this hypothetical starting point is established, we can then select a specific preference ranking. And it is only then that we can bring the values and ethical orientations—historically defined—that make us lean toward a certain conception of justice, a specific idea of redistribution, a given idea of the good.

In a nutshell, then, when we decide we cannot refuse to take information into account. And when we reflect on choices we must also be prepared to observe the opposite route:

> What is, in contrast, indispensably important is an adequate understanding of the informational basis of evaluation—the kind of information we need to examine in order to assess what is going on and what is being seriously neglected.
>
> (Sen, 1999, p. 286)

Paying attention to the information that supports value judgments should help establish the fact that the informational basis of these judgments must always be identified, and it must thus be possible submit them to continual forms of validation through public discussion.

We started by asking whether knowledge helps us to decide, and we have now come to the point where we can begin to formulate an answer. Demoting rationality does not mean embracing weak thought, since it is in any case important that procedures be put in place (though how they are actually used is another matter) for collecting and comparing ideas and information about choices that have public repercussions. One aspect that remains to be unpacked, however, is that of how choices are communicated. Starting from different decision-making models, what forms can communication take?

8 Uncertain choices and public justification

Once we have agreed that collecting information is necessary, the problem of choice must still be solved. Decisions, in fact, ripen in particular organizational environments that influence both the models of choice and the resulting communication strategies (Boltanski & Thévenot, 1991; Tilly, 2006). And the problems are not limited to deciding what information is needed to make a fully informed choice of the routes that should be taken, given that—as we mentioned earlier—these routes are not always well posted. In the case of the current pandemic, for example, even if the institutions do not have all the information that would be needed to start phase 2 of reopening, they are nevertheless required to make decisions in this connection and find appropriate ways of explaining them to the public, doing so in a way that does not further destabilize a situation that is already an acute social emergency. The need to justify choices is thus burdened by ambivalence: choices are based on unavoidably incomplete information, and their outcomes are often uncertain, but the public must be quickly convinced that they are credible and rigorous. One way to avoid the paradoxes that this entails is to fall back on secrecy (to which we will return in the following chapter), presenting the public with the facts without troubling to explain the rationale for the choices that were made, but this approach runs counter to the obligation to provide the transparency that is widely expected of the institutions. However, trying to be clear about the processes behind the choices is often unrealistic because of the inherent uncertainty that the actors must navigate. Consequently, it may be that "collections of choices" and "collections of opinions" are coupled virtually at random as posited in the so-called *garbage can model* (March & Olsen, 1976; March, 1988). This model of organizational choice is particularly attuned to problems involving uncertainty, time pressures and difficulties in offering scientific proof. The solution to be adopted is decided—again, almost at random—from a set of options that are all more or less applicable, but whose implications we are unable to assess. Here too, this involves a species of rational choice, albeit one stemming from an organizational rationality which is based on the need to act and is almost independent, in this case, of the link between the problem and the adopted solution:

> ... choosing a "solution" is in any case useful even if it does not match any of the problems at hand, but postpones them, diverts them, moves them elsewhere. The problem being tackled, the type of solution adopted, are mere details compared to the fact of having made a decision, of having extricated ourselves from the impasse, of reasserting our ability to manoeuvre in a given situation.
>
> (Negri, 1995, p. 16)

The "garbage can" model corresponds to a style of communication that tends to seek ex-post legitimation for decisions that were made—as we said—almost at random. Had this "randomness" been clear, it would have undermined the idea that public opinion has public decision-makers. Consequently, communication's task in this is to create a consistent image of organizational processes after the fact. There is a risk, however, of communicating more in order to make the decisions acceptable than to facilitate access by the public and stakeholders and to involve them in the decision-making process.

At the opposite extreme, the *synoptic rationality model* is based on unrealistic expectations of having all necessary information, examining it exhaustively and then choosing the best prospect. In this case, the task of public justification is to make people understand which interpretation of the law and regulations adopted by the administration is the best, i.e., the most objective possible. Communicating and justifying the routes that have been taken help boost the climate of security instilled by choosing to pursue clear, certain norms and values as part of a process that takes place in a shared, stable domain of meanings and that participates in disseminating those that are most in line with the rules that are to be applied.

In both models, the role of public communication is one of symbolic integration whose "purpose is to convey the values that characterize and drive each institution" (Mancini, 1999, p. 116). The goal is essentially to preserve the system's stability by legitimating—in the case of the synoptic rationality model—the interpretation of the rules that is considered most correct and, in the garbage can model, the existence of the institutions as such.

The garbage can and synoptic rationality models by no means account for the full range of models of choice, but are the two poles of a continuum. A further pair of models lying midway between these poles is frequently mentioned in the politico-administrative literature (Bobbio, 1994, 1996) and poses different problems in terms of the forms of communication they require. We will now look at both briefly.

The *cognitive model* fully acknowledges the uncertainty in which choice takes place. It sees uncertainty as a constitutive feature, not only of the world, but also of each of the individuals and collective actors who participate in the decision-making process. To cope with it, the actors tend to rely on forms of procedural rationality, employing "schemes of explanation that have already worked in similar situations. The solution is found by analogy or similarity and depends on whether interpretive frames are available" (Bobbio, 1996, p. 27). However, using forms of procedural rationality—because of the tendency to draw on approaches similar to those that have already been used—may not be sufficient to address questions that put institutions up against problems that are radically different from anything they have ever faced before.

For this model, public communication seeks to link the actors' cognitive models to the conceptual frameworks they use to interpret reality and select the aspects they consider important. Here the power to choose is far less centralized than in the rational choice model. Consequently, communication between the different organizational units that make choices when collecting, transmitting and processing information is crucial, as is how each actor defines the problems and selects the alternatives for that unit. As Bobbio tells us:

> [T]he choices of a ministry or a municipal administration cannot be explained only by considering the interests or the intentions of the political figures involved (the minister, the mayor or the council members); the latter, in fact, are influenced by how the various offices define the problems and choose between alternatives, on the basis of consolidated methods that tend to persist over time.
>
> (1996, p. 30)

The cognitive model emphasizes the importance of representing problems as the only way of solving them: "solving a problem simply means representing it so as to make the solution transparent" (Simon, 1996, p. 132). Consequently, "much problem solving effort is directed at structuring problems, and only a fraction of it at solving problems once they are structured" (Simon, 1973, in Bobbio, 1996, p. 28). From this standpoint, institutional communication—within each organization and between different organizations—contributes to how arguments are formulated, priorities are selected and the public policy agenda is set.

The last model is the *incremental model*, where public communication's goal is to make up for the fragmentation of actors that the model assumes. We have said that in the cognitive model, uncertainty arises from the limitations of each actor involved, who thus tends to employ concepts similar to those used in the past. Here, by contrast, uncertainty is connected to the fact that "decisions are always—to some extent—the outcome of collective processes" (Bobbio, 1996, p. 31). Since the uncertainty of the decision depends on the fragmentation of the actors involved in the process, communication's task is to clarify what ends can be chosen given the available means. Practical applications of the model have included such techniques as *alternative dispute resolution*, which seek to build consensus among the actors through mediation practices. The point that concerns us here is that "in these models the public interest is not determined beforehand, but springs from consensual negotiation between the parties in question" (Susskind & Cruikshank, 1987, in Bobbio, 1996, p. 38).

This short summary of the models and forms that communication can take in each area of decision-making sought to provoke thought about the connections between information, choices and the *responsible* use of the ways choices are communicated to the public. The constraints and resources for the forms of communication that can be employed in interactions between participants in the decision-making process are established by the organizational context, and it is thus important to be aware of them. However, this does not mean that the decisions made in complex processes or organizational milieux, where an increasing number of actors have a say, can be explained via simplified pictures of reality, even if such pictures can help pinpoint particular problems in the processes in question. With the story of Annapurna, we drew attention to the fact that she does not try to deny complexity but seeks feasible—and *responsible*—ways to arrive at a well-thought-out decision. Being responsible means finding ways to bring uncertainty into the equation, without waiting until it can be eliminated. Responsibility in the dynamics of communication thus entails being aware of the increasing weight that words take on in rapidly changing contexts where tensions abound (Butler, 1997; Melucci, 2000; Bourdieu & Wacquant, 2001) and reckoning with public communication's crucial role in defining what for each of us can be considered "normal" or "right". As Melucci argued, "Whatever categories are introduced, we must be conscious of the fact that they are not neutral as regards the effects they produce" (2000, p. 20). But what happens when there are not enough resources to go around? How does the need for rationing tie in with the images of a safeguarded public that healthcare systems should project? These and other aspects of the images of health will be addressed in the following chapter.

Notes

1 In addition to the data from the WHO report, the sources included a series of general population surveys conducted by the Eurobarometer in 15 European countries between April and May 1998, and two surveys conducted at the end of 2000 by the Harvard School of Public Health in Canada and in the United States (Blendon et al., 2001, p. 13).

2 Transparency International is a nongovernmental organization that each year measures the state of corruption in 180 countries around the world. The index ranks each country by its perceived level of public sector corruption, drawing on 13 data sources which range from nepotism in the civil service, to the government's ability to enforce integrity mechanisms and to legal protection for journalists, investigators and whistleblowers.

3 Merton defines a self-fulfilling prophecy as "a *false* definition of the situation evoking a new behavior which makes the originally false definition of the situation come *true*" (1968, p. 477).

4 The "best to best" principle, where more resources are allocated to those who are considered best, has nothing inevitable about it. Resources could be allocated in equal shares, or it could be decided to give more to those who are in greatest difficulty ("best to worst"). See Bevan & Hood, 2006, p. 6. As we will see in the conclusions to this chapter, the nature of the information is often not helpful even when it is clear which approach will be taken.

5 The Foundational Economy is a concept stemming from the work of Karel Williams and the University of Manchester's Centre for Research on Socio-Cultural Change (CRESC), which has assembled an international research group that investigates the characteristics of the economic space as they relate to the needs of a particular community. The basic assumption is that "the foundational economy must serve the community, rather than using the community as a pool of resources to be extracted" (Barbera et al., 2016, p. IX).

6 In response to the statement, "Knowing that mortality statistics will be made public influences your decision on whether to intervene in critical ill patients with high
   expected mortality rates", 31.7% of participants stated that they agree, and 47.5%
   stated that they strongly agree (Narins et al., 2005, p. 85).
7 INPS responded to criticisms by stating that performance as regards revoking disability benefits was evaluated at the regional level and that individual physicians were thus
   not able to influence the final amount of their compensation. Apart from individual
   interests, the outcome in this case is limited to shifting the gaming mechanisms from
   the level of individual physicians to that of the regions, which does nothing to resolve
   the ambiguity of indicators that take a favorable view of cutting benefits for certain
   categories of patient.
8 In this connection, Elster (1983) speaks of adaptive preference formation or adaptive
   preference change. This mechanism can, as in the fable of the fox and the grapes, lead us
   to emphasize the negative attributes of the option that is not available to us (we decide we
   do not want the grapes, not because we cannot reach them, but because they are sour).
9 Between late March and early April 2020, the Italian Central Anticrime Directorate,
   an arm of the National Police and the Ministry of the Interior, warned of the need
   for vigilance in fragile sectors that were most affected by the pandemic measures in
   order to prevent corruption and infiltration in public contracts and healthcare. In fact,
   there were a number of documented instances of profiteering, ranging from sales of
   disinfectants and personal protective equipment at wildly inflated prices, to full-scale
   scams. On April 3, for example, the country's anti-adulteration and health units (Nuclei
   Anti Sofisticazione, NAS), shut down a number of websites selling ordinary dietary
   supplements at enormous markups, extolling their supposedly miraculous power to
   prevent COVID-19.
10 According to the OECD (2017), wasteful spending mainly occurs when patients do not
   receive the right care, benefits could be obtained with fewer resources or resources are
   unnecessarily taken away from patient care.
11 D.F. Thompson, founder of the Harvard University Center for Ethics and the Pro-
   fessions, defines a conflict of interest as "a set of conditions in which professional
   judgment concerning a primary interest (such as a patient's welfare or the validity
   of research) tends to be unduly influenced by a secondary interest (such as financial
   gain)" (1993, quoted in Dirindin et al., 2018, p. 13).
12 On April 10, 2020, a press release by the president of the GIMBE Foundation decried
   a misleading use of the data on recovered patients by the regional administration of
   Lombardia. He referred specifically to 15,706 cases which the administration recorded
   as "self-isolating" in the column headed "Discharged/Recovered", which were thus
   added to the number of "Total Recovered". Most other regional governments use
   the clinical and virological recovery criteria established by the Technical Scientific
   Committee.
   As the president emphasized, overestimating the number of recovered patients gives
   the public a false idea of how the pandemic is progressing and influences political and
   health decisions.
   www.gimbe.org/pagine/341/it/comunicati-stampa
13 An earlier version of the last two sections of the chapter was published in the conclusions of the book *Dilemmi del welfare* (Bosco, 2002).
14 Cinema and literature have also dealt for some time with the ambivalent relationship
   between risk and control. From this standpoint, the films of Luis Buñuel (1962's *The
   Exterminating Angel,* for example) have been illuminating, as are the novels of J. C.
   Ballard—*High-Rise* (1975); *Running High* (1988)—which explore contexts where the
   desire to keep insecurity in check gradually degenerates into the construction of life-
   worlds dominated by chaos and the complete absence of hope.

15 Springing from the difficulty of accepting that we inhabit worlds that are outside our control, the idea of the "risk society" has garnered increasing attention in the social sciences. The expression *Risikogesellschaft* was coined by Ulrich Beck in a celebrated text that appeared in 1986. Beck and a number of other scholars have returned to the theme of risk and its social implications at the macro and micro levels in subsequent years (see *inter alia* Beck, 2000; Giddens, 1990, Ranci, 1997, Bauman, 1998, 1999a, 1999b; Luhmann, 1991; Castel, 2003, 2016).
16 In addition to the one we deal with in detail, Sen presents, and refutes, two other forms of skepticism: the first holds that given the heterogeneity of preferences and values in a given society, it is not possible to have a coherent framework for reasoned social assessment. The second doubts that it is possible to agree on a broader range of values and behavioral norms that go at all beyond ubiquitous human selfishness and self-interest (1999).
17 Procedural rationality defined by Simon (1985), as Bobbio notes, is "directed towards adapting the means to rules and procedures that are largely predetermined, even if they are continually corrected on the basis of individual or organizational experience" (1996, p. 27).
18 The need to learn from what we are doing creates a need for information, making learning an essential part of evaluation. Learning can take place by observing the consequences (positive or negative, predictable or unpredictable) of any given action and by attempting to identify the causal links that made the action possible (Martini & Cais, 1999).

References

Adam, B. (1999). *La responsabilità e la dimensione temporale della scienza, della tecnologia e della natura*. In Leccardi, C. (Ed.), *Limiti della modernità. Trasformazioni del mondo e della conoscenza*. Roma: Carocci.
Agnoletto, V. (2018). Inps: più prestazioni revochi e più guadagni. Una proposta inaccettabile per un medico. *IlFattoQuotidiano.it*/BLOG di Vittorio Agnoletto, 9 October.
Ballard, J. C. (1975). *High-Rise*. London: Jonathan Cape Ltd.
Ballard, J. C. (1988). *Running Wild*. London: Hutchinson.
Barbera, F., Dagnes, J., Salento, A., & Spina, F. (Eds.). (2016). *Il capitale quotidiano. Un manifesto per l'economia fondamentale*. Roma: Donzelli Editore.
Bauman, Z. (1998). *Globalization: The Human Consequences*. Cambridge: Polity Press.
Bauman, Z. (1999a). *La società dell'incertezza*. Bologna: il Mulino.
Bauman, Z. (1999b). *In Search of Politics*. Cambridge: Polity Press.
Beck, T. R. (1830). Statistical Notices of Some of the Lunatic Asylums in the United States. *Transactions of the Albany Institute, 1*(1), 60–83.
Beck, U. (1986). *Risikogesellschaft Auf dem Weg in eine andere Moderne*. Frankfurt: Suhrkamp. English translation by M. Ritter (1992), *Risk Society: Towards a New Modernity*. London: SAGE Publications Ltd.
Beck, U. (2000). *Freiheit oder Kapitalismus: Gesellschaft neu denken*. Frankfurt: Suhrkamp. trad. it *Libertà o capitalismo? Varcare la soglia della modernità*. Roma: Carocci, 2001.
Berger, P., & Luckmann, T. (1995). *Modernity, Pluralism and the Crisis of Meaning: The Orientation of Modern Man*. Gütersloch: Bertelsmann Stiftung.
Berman, E. P., & Hirschman, D. (2018). The Sociology of Quantification: Where Are We Now? *Contemporary Sociology, 47*(3), 257–266. https://doi.org/10.1177/0094306118767649.
Bevan, G., & Hood, C. (2006). What's Measured Is What Matters: Targets and Gaming in the English Public Health System. *Public Administration, 84*, 517–538. https://doi.org/10.1111/j.1467-9299.2006.00600.x.

Blendon, R. J., Kim, M., & Benson, J. M. (2001). The Public Versus the World Health Organization on Health System Performance. *Health Affairs, 20*(3), 10–20. https://doi.org/10.1377/hlthaff.20.3.10.

Bobbio, L. (1994). *Di questo accordo lieto. Sulla risoluzione negoziale dei conflitti ambientali*. Torino: Rosenberg & Sellier.

Bobbio, L. (1996). *La democrazia non abita a Gordio. Studio dei processi decisionali politico-amministrativi*. Milano: Franco Angeli.

Bobbio, M. (2004). *Giuro di esercitare la medicina in libertà e indipendenza*. Torino: Einaudi.

Bobbio, M. (2017). *Troppa medicina. Un uso eccessivo può nuocere alla salute*. Torino: Einaudi.

Boltanski, L., & Thévenot, L. (1991). *De la justification. Les économies de la grandeur*. Paris: Édition Gallimard. English translation by Catherine Porter (2006), *On Justification. Economies of Worth*. Princeton: Princeton University Press.

Borghi, V. (2019). The Possible in the Real: Infrastructures of Experience, Cosmopolitanism from Below and Sociology. *Quaderni di Teoria Sociale, 1*, 35–60. www.morlacchilibri.com/universitypress/allegati/QTS_1_2019.pdf.

Borghi, V., & Giullari, B. (2015). Real Abstractions and Sociological Imagination. Transformations of Informational Basis, Social Practices and Horizons of Research. *Rassegna Italiana di Sociologia, 3–4*, 379–404. https://doi.org/10.1423/81797.

Bosco, N. (2002). *Dilemmi del Welfare. Politiche assistenziali e comunicazione pubblica*. Milano: Edizioni Angelo Guerini.

Bosco, N. (2006). La drosofila e altre storie: ovvero dell'incontro tra normalità e certezza. *Meridiana, 55*, 125–140.

Bourdieu, P., & Wacquant, E. L. (2001). Neoliberal Newspeak: Notes on the New Planetary Vulgate. *Radical Philosophy, 105*, 1–6.

Burawoy, M. (2005). For Public Sociology. *American Sociological Review, 70*(1), 4–26. https://doi.org/10.1177/000312240507000102.

Busso, S. (2015). "What Works". On Effectiveness and Quantification in Changing Social Policies. *Rassegna Italiana di Sociologia, 3–4*, 479–502. https://doi.org/10.1423/81802.

Butler, J. (1997). *Excitable Speech. A Politics of the Performative*. London: Routledge.

Canduro, A. (2018). *Big Pharma e la privatizzazione del Sistema Sanitario Nazionale*. Sbilanciamoci Info/org. http://sbilanciamoci.info/big-pharma-e-la-privatizzazione-dei-ssn/.

Canguilhem, G. (1966). *Le normal et le pathologique*. Paris: Presses Universitaires de France. English translation by Carolyn R. Fawcett, & Robert S. Cohen (1978), *On the Normal and the Pathological*. Dordrecht: D. Reidal Publishing.

Carraro, F., & Quezel, M. (2018). *Salute S.p.A. La sanità svenduta alle assicurazioni: il racconto di due insider*. Milano: Chiarelettere editore srl.

Cartabellotta, N., Cottafava, E., Luceri, R., Mosti, M., & Orsi, F. (2018). *Il Servizio Sanitario Nazionale nelle classifiche internazionali*. Report Osservatorio GIMBE, n.4/2018, September. www.gimbe.org/osservatorio/Report_Osservatorio_GIMBE_2018.04_Classifiche_SSN.pdf.

Castel, R. (2003). *L'insécurité sociale: Qu'est ce qu'être protégé?* Paris: Seuil.

Castel, R. (2016). The Rise of Uncertainties. *Critical Horizons, 17*(2), 160–167. https://doi.org/10.1080/14409917.2016.1153886.

Commission for Health Improvement. (2003). *What CHI has found in: Ambulance trusts*. London: The Stationery Office. http://www.healthcarecommission.org.uk/NationalFindings/NationalThemedReports/Ambulance/fs/en

Cooley, A., & Snyder, J. (2015). Rank Has Its Privileges: How International Ratings Dumb Down Global Governance. *Foreign Affairs*, *94*(6), 101–108. https://heinonline.org/HOL/Page?collection=journals&handle=hein.journals/fora94&id=1351&men_tab=srchresults.

De Leonardis, O. (2001). *Le istituzioni. Come e perché parlarne*. Milano: Carocci.

Desrosières, A. (1998). *The Politics of Large Numbers: A History of Statistical Reasoning*. Cambridge, MA: Harvard University Press.

Dirindin, N., Rivoiro, C., & De Fiore, L. (2018). *Conflitti di interesse e salute. Come industrie e istituzioni condizionano le scelte del medico*. Bologna: il Mulino.

Elster, J. (1983). *Sour Grapes. Studies in the Subversion of Rationality*. Cambridge: Cambridge University Press.

Elster, J. (1997). *Razionalità, Enciclopedia delle Scienze Sociali*, Vol. VII. Roma: Istituto della Enciclopedia Italiana Treccani, 230–241.

Espeland, W. N., & Sauder, M. (2007). Rankings and Reactivity: How Public Measures Recreate Social Worlds. *American Journal of Sociology*, *113*(1), 1–40. https://doi.org/10.1086/517897.

Esposito, E., & Stark, D. (2019). What's Observed in a Rating? Rankings as Orientation in the Face of Uncertainty. *Theory, Culture & Society*, *36*(4), 3–26. https://doi.org/10.1177/0263276419826276.

Fabbri, A., Gregoraci, G., Tedesco, D., Ferretti, F., Gilardi, F., Iemmi, D., . . . Rinaldi, A. (2016). Conflict of Interest Between Professional Medical Societies and Industry: A Cross-Sectional Study of Italian Medical Societies' Websites. *British Medical Journal Open*, *6*, e011124. https://doi.org/10.1136/bmjopen-2016-011124.

Ferraris, M. (2017). *Postverità e altri enigmi*. Bologna: il Mulino.

Festinger, L. (1957). *A Theory of Cognitive Dissonance*. Stanford, CA: Stanford University Press.

Foucault, M. (1985/1998). Life: Experience and Science. In Rabinow, P. (Ed.), *The Essential Works of Michel Foucault 1954–1984*, Vol. 2. New York: The New Press.

Foucault, M. (1999). *Les Anormaux. Cours au collège de France. 1974–1975*. Paris: Seuil/Gallimard. English translation by Graham Burchell (2003), *Abnormal. Lectures at the Collége de France, 1974–1975*. London and New York: Verso.

Foucault, M. (2012). *Du Gouvernment des Vivants. Cours au Collège de France 1979–1980*. Paris: Éditions Gallimard. English translation by Graham Burchell (2014), *On the Government of the Living. Lectures at the Collége de France, 1979–1980*. New York: Palgrave Macmillan.

Frey, B. S. (1997). *Not Just for the Money: An Economic Theory of Personal Motivation*. Cheltenham: Edward Elgar Publishing.

Gakidou, E., Murray, C., & Frank, J. (2000). *Measuring Preferences on Health System Performance Assessment*. GPE Discussion Paper Series No. 20. Geneva: World Health Organization. www.who.int/healthinfo/paper20.pdf.

Garattini, S., & Bertelé, V. (2007). Non-Inferiority Trials Are Unethical Because They Disregard Patients' Interests. *Lancet*, *370*. http://doi.org/10.1016/S0140-6736(07)61604-3.

Giddens, A. (1990). *The Consequences of Modernity*. Cambridge: Polity Press.

Gobbi, B. (2016). *L'accusa di Cantone: sanità terreno di scorribanda per delinquenti di ogni risma*. ilSole24ore, 6 April. https://st.ilsole24ore.com/art/notizie/2016-04-06/l-accusa-cantone-sanita-terreno-scorribanda-delinquenti-ogni-risma-110445.shtml?uuid=AC3A721C.

Greenhalgh, T., Howick, J., Maskrey, N., & Evidence Based Medicine Renaissance Group. (2014). Evidence Based Medicine: A Movement in Crisis? *British Medical Journal (Clinical Research ed.)*, *348*, g3725. https://doi.org/10.1136/bmj.g3725.

Hill, A., Simmons, B., Gotham, D., & Fortunak, J. (2016). Rapid Reductions in Prices for Generic Sofosbuvir and Daclatasvir to Treat Hepatitis C. *Journal of Virus Eradication*, *2*(1), 28–31. www.ncbi.nlm.nih.gov/pmc/articles/PMC4946692/.

Lanzara, G. F. (1993). *Capacità negativa. Competenza progettuale e modelli di intervento nelle organizzazioni*. Bologna: il Mulino. Roma: Carocci.

LeGrand, J. (2003). *Motivation, Agency and Public Policy*. Oxford: Oxford University Press.

Luhmann, N. (1991). *Sociologie des Risikos*. Berlin: de Gruyter. English translation by Rhodes Barrett (1993), *Risk: A Sociological Theory*. New York: Aldine de Gruyter.

Mancini, P. (1999). *Manuale di comunicazione pubblica*. Bari: Editori Laterza.

March, J. G. (1988). *Decisions and Organizations*. Oxford: Basil Blackwell Ltd.

March, J. G., & Olsen, J. P. (1976). *Ambiguity and Choice in Organizations*. Bergen: Universitetsforlaget.

Martini, A., & Cais, G. (1999). *Controllo (di gestione) e valutazione (delle politiche): un (ennesimo ma non ultimo) tentativo di sistemazione concettuale*. Paper presented at the Second Congress of Associazione Italiana Valutazione, 15–17 April, Naples.

Melucci, A. (2000). *Parole chiave. Per un nuovo lessico delle scienze sociali*. Roma: Carocci.

Merton, R. K. (1968). *Social Theory and Social Structure*. New York: The Free Press.

Narins, C. R., Dozier, A. M., Ling, F. S., & Zareba, W. (2005). The Influence of Public Reporting of Outcome Data on Medical Decision Making by Physicians. *Archives of Internal Medicine*, *165*(1), 83–87. https://doi.org/10.1001/archinte.165.1.83.

Navarro, P. (2008). The MBA Core Curricula of Top-Ranked U.S. Business Schools: A Study in Failure? *Academy of Management Learning & Education*, *7*(1), 108–123. https://doi.org/10.5465/amle.2008.31413868.

Negri, N. (1995). Dal Rumore alle difficoltà. In *Ires, Atteggiamenti e comportamenti verso gli immigrati in alcuni ambienti istituzionali*. Torino: Rosenberg & Sellier.

Noto, G., Belardi, P., & Vainieri, M. (2020). Unintended Consequences of Expenditure Targets on Resource Allocation in Health Systems. *Health Policy*, *124*(4), 462–469. https://doi.org/10.1016/j.healthpol.2020.01.012.

OECD. (2017). *Tackling Wasteful Spending on Health*. Paris: OECD Publishing. www.oecd.org/health/tackling-wasteful-spending-on-health-9789264266414-en.htm.

Pitch, T. (2001). Relativo all'occidente. *il Manifesto*, 3 October.

Pizzorno, A. (2007). *Il velo della diversità: Studi su razionalità e riconoscimento*. Milano: Feltrinelli.

Porter, T. M. (1995). *Trust in Numbers: The Pursuit of Objectivity in Science and Public Life*. Princeton: Princeton University Press.

Porter, T. M. (2003). Measurement, Objectivity, and Trust. *Measurement: Interdisciplinary Research and Perspectives*, *1*(4), 241–255. https://doi.org/10.1207/S15366359MEA0104_1.

Porter, T. M. (2012). Funny Numbers. *Journal of Current Cultural Research*, *4*, 595–598. www.cultureunbound.ep.liu.se/v4/a32/cu12v4a32.pdf.

Pritchard, J. C. (1835). *A Treatise on Insanity and Other Disorders Affecting the Mind*. London: Sherwood, Gilbert, & Piper.

Ranci, C. (1997). *La società del rischio. Vulnerabilità ed esclusione sociale in Lombardia*. Milano: Guerini e Associati.

Rao, H. (1994). The Social Construction of Reputation: Certification Contests, Legitimation, and the Survival of Organizations in the American Automobile Industry: 1895–1912. *Strategic Management Journal*, *15*, 29–44. https://doi.org/10.1002/smj.4250150904.

Re, A. (2015). La centralità di una Comunità Scientifica Allargata. In Re, A., Callari, T. C., & Occelli, C. (Eds.), *Sfide attuali, passate, future. Il percorso di Ivar Oddone.* Torino: Otto Editore, 15–22.

Report Curiamo la corruzione. (2017). https://healthworks.ti-health.org/projects/curiamo-la-corruzione-we-treat-corruption/.

Ricolfi, L. (2020). E se il Covid-19 fosse già dilagato anche al Sud? *HumePage*, 8 April. www.fondazionehume.it/societa/e-se-il-covid-19-fosse-gia-dilagato-anche-al-sud/.

Rindova, V. P., Martins, L. L., Srinivas, S. B., & Chandler, B. (2018). The Good, the Bad, and the Ugly of Organizational Rankings; A Multidisciplinary Review of the Literature and Directions for Future Research. *Journal of Management*, *44*(6), 2175–2208. https://doi.org/10.1177%2F0149206317741962.

Rubin, R. S., & Dierdorff, E. C. (2009). How Relevant Is the MBA? Assessing the Alignment of Required Curricula and Required Managerial Competencies. *Academy of Management Learning & Education*, *8*(2), 208–224. https://doi.org/10.5465/amle.2009.41788843.

Sánchez, F. J., Sotorrío, L. L., & Baraibar Díez, E. (2012). Can Corporate Reputation Protect Companies' Value? Spanish Evidence of the 2007 Financial Crash. *Corporate Reputation Review*, *15*, 228–239. https://doi.org/10.1057/crr.2012.13.

Schütte, S., Acevedo, P., & Flahault, A. (2018). Health Systems Around the World—A Comparison of Existing Health System Rankings. *Journal of Global Health*, *8*(1), 010407. https://doi.org/10.7189/jogh.08.010407.

Sen, A. K. (1982). *Choice, Welfare and Measurement.* Oxford: Blackwell.

Sen, A. K. (1987). *On Ethics and Economics.* Oxford: Basil Blackwell.

Sen, A. K. (1999). *Development as Freedom.* New York: Alfred A. Knopf, Inc.

Simmel, G. (1971). *On Individuality and Social Forms.* Edited by D. N. Levine. Chicago: Chicago University Press.

Simon, H. A. (1973). The Structure of Ill Structured Problems. *Artificial Intelligence*, 181–201. https://cschan.public.iastate.edu/235/6_Simon_Ill_defined_problem.pdf.

Simon, H. A. (1985). Human Nature in Politics: The Dialogue of Psychology with Political Science. *American Political Science Review*, *79*(2), 293–320. www.jstor.org/stable/1956650.

Simon, H. A. (1996). *The Sciences of the Artificial.* Cambridge, MA: MIT Press.

Supiot, A. (2015). De l'harmonie par le calcul à la gouvernance par les nombres. *Rassegna Italiana di Sociologia, 3–4*, 455–464. https://doi.org/10.1423/81800.

Susskind, L., & Cruikshank, J. (1987). *Breaking the Impasse. Consensual Approaches to Resolving Public Disputes.* New York: Basic Books.

Thompson, D. F. (1993). Understanding Financial Conflicts of Interest. *The New England Journal of Medicine*, *329*(8), 573–576. https://doi.org/10.1056/NEJM199308193290812.

Tilly, C. (2006). *Why? What Happens When People Give Reasons . . . and Why.* Princeton: Princeton University Press.

Weber, M. (1922). *Wirtschaft und Gesellschaft: Grundriss der verstehenden Soziologie,* 2 vol., Tübingen. English translation by Ephraim Fischoff (1978), *Economy and Society. An Outline of Interpretive Sociology,* Roth, G., & Wittich, C. (Eds.). Berkeley: University of California Press.

WHO. (2000). The World Health Report 2000. *Press Release*, 21 June. www.who.int/whr/2000/en/press_release.htm.

Zerubavel, E. (2018). *Taken for Granted. The Remarkable Power of the Unremarkable.* Princeton: Princeton University Press.

Chapter 3

Rationing and communication ambiguities

At the end of the 1980s, the state of Oregon decided to rethink the criteria governing public access to its healthcare system. The idea was to find additional resources to fund public health in a system like that in the United States, where health is not considered a right, and the programs available for those who cannot afford any form of insurance coverage (because they do not have regular employment, for example) are marginal at best. Pursuing the goal of extending access to healthcare to more people called for a careful reckoning of costs and benefits, in line with the utilitarian approach that, in its most general shape, seeks to maximize benefits in a given community. Choosing not to provide public funding for certain extremely expensive procedures, for example, would have made it possible to use the savings to extend free basic health coverage to a larger number of indigent people. Thus, if the organ transplant program were not state-funded, the amount of money needed for only 34 transplants would have covered healthcare for 1500 low-income people (Vineis & Capri, 1994, pp. 98–99). At first sight, the argument undeniably holds water. But imagining an abstract situation that sets the benefits of the few against those of the many is one thing, while replacing the numbers with real people—and their stories, fears, fragilities and needs—is quite another. And so, when a seven-year-old boy dies because he was denied a bone marrow transplant, the full implications of this approach suddenly become far clearer and harder to swallow than they seemed at first, and battle lines inevitably form in a bitter debate on the approach's iniquity.[1]

Discussing principles, in fact, is not easy, and can be even more complicated when choices can lead to outcomes that are virtually impossible to bring into the equation beforehand: homing in on a single case, as the criticisms of the model adopted in Oregon would seem to demand, does not always yield the hoped-for results and, lacking a clear common goal, there is always a very real risk of driving an even wider wedge between opposing viewpoints and approaches. In this connection, Klein & Maybin tell us of the case of a ten-year-old girl—Jaymee Bowen—diagnosed with a recurrence of acute myeloid leukemia. A bone marrow transplant had not worked, and the physicians had advised against further chemotherapy and a second transplant, "given the pain and the discomfort involved, and the low chances of success" (2012, p. 7). As Ham and Pickard (1998) note, the

DOI: 10.4324/9780367854515-4

family opposed interrupting treatment, and a long, painful legal battle ensued, much heightened by media coverage. An anonymous donor provided funds so that the child could receive a costly experimental treatment, but, after some initial respite, Jaymee died less than a year later.

These two episodes testify to the objective difficulties to be encountered in the territory we are venturing into, and are an invitation to prudence in weighing choices and trying to predict their outcomes. But venture we will, one step at a time.

As we mentioned earlier, it is not easy to decide what criteria should be used to make choices that hinge on a range of considerations about justice, healthcare providers' ethics and patients' quality of life or even their survival. Criticisms of the utilitarian approach emphasize, for example, that if we do not consider fairness of treatment in relation to the wellbeing of each and every patient, we cannot expect there to be anything even remotely resembling a right to healthcare. The risk, as the opponents of the utilitarian model maintain, is that assigning greater importance to the benefits that a certain allocation of resources can bring for the community at the expense of its outcome for individual patients can increase inequalities in access to care. For example, one of the risks of prioritizing a cost–benefit approach is that severely ill patients may be systematically denied resources that are available to others, given that:

> They cost society much more than they are able to produce, and maximizing their wellbeing undoubtedly conflicts with maximizing utility for the group.
> (Buchanan, 1989, in Vineis & Capri, 1994, p. 97)

Consequently, deciding that the benefits to the community outweigh those to the individual makes it difficult to recognize that severely disabled people and patients with complex conditions which often require costly treatments have a right to care. And it is hard not to be repelled by a point of view that would seem to be at odds with values that are deeply rooted in the idea that many people have of society: that of solidarity, for example, and protecting the weakest, or of the veil of ignorance (see Chapter 1), whereby embracing the need for a universalistic and inclusive conception of rights does not even require that we believe in solidarity, given that we cannot predict what will happen to us in the future and can thus hope that publicly funded care options will be available to the most fragile members of society, since we might end up needing them ourselves.

1 A grim calculus? The implications of rationing based on economic considerations

Early in April 2020, *The Economist* printed a leader on the grim calculus involved in the tradeoff between saving human lives with lockdown policies that reduce the number of hospitalized patients and deaths and saving the economy by allowing businesses to reopen.

Not all economists agree on how the costs and benefits work out for the different options, nor does the statistical value assigned to a human life appear in their ever-so-confident analyses: while the average figure quoted in the United States is about 14.5 million dollars for a life, some sources maintain this sum should be cut by around 37% for the elderly (bringing the figure down to 9 million), whereas others put a value of just 3.7 million dollars on the over-seventies (Feltri, 2020). These are figures that can seem arid and, in certain respects, a bit disconcerting, but over and above that fact, the issues they raise deserve careful consideration. How, for instance, can we answer the following questions? "Some unemployment and bankruptcy is a price worth paying, but how much? If extreme social distancing fails to stop the disease, how long should it persist?".[2]

For some time now, approaches that set collective benefits—like the number of lives saved or years of life gained, or savings in the cost of treatment—against the wellbeing of individual people have fueled controversy. A decade or so ago, the then 84-year-old philosopher Mary Warnock drew a barrage of criticism when she stated that dementia sufferers were an excessive burden on their families and Britain's National Health Service, and that it would thus be morally acceptable—and in her opinion better—to help those who did not want to be a weight on others or were in fact considered as such to end their own lives (Beckford, 2008). Though her words caused widespread shock at the time, we cannot deny that there is still a highly stigmatizing view of dementia and similar conditions that accepts individuals and their identities only if they are rational and fully functioning (Batsch et al., 2012). If the prevailing idea is that our value as human beings depends on some ideal version of how we function, the burden of care for many who suffer from these conditions becomes unacceptable. According to Peter Kevern, when faced with complex diseases, we are made to choose what lives deserve respect and who is entitled to say what they are worth:

> Dementia forces us to choose. Confronted with someone who can no longer think or remember clearly, who cannot conceptualise a range of options or contribute to the productivity of material society, we are forced to decide whether we will accept them as a person or not.
>
> (2017, p. 2)

Responding to these demands is not easy, and the idea that being a valuable human being means having a full command of rational thought and coherent memory and the opposing notion that autonomy and fragility are intrinsic facets of the human condition have vied with each other in all cultures and throughout history. It is not so long ago, for example—though the memory has perhaps faded—that a warped understanding of the theories of positive eugenics (which sought to increase the proliferation of desirable traits in a given population) provided a pseudoscientific alibi for the genocides perpetrated by Europe's totalitarian regimes under the banner of racial purity (De Stefano, 2008).

But even without bringing such extremes into the picture, the debate sparked by the dilemmas that arise from differing conceptions of justice and fairness and how they should be tackled, as well as the value to be assigned to different forms of life and the many characteristics that make up the human condition, has been intense even if it has chiefly played out in rather restricted circles. As we will see, wider-ranging discussions—those involving the public, for example—have been fairly rare, precisely because of the difficulties in framing and grasping the implications of such complex issues which, once raised, impel some sort of response from the institutions.

For example, a specific subsector of ethics known as "trolleyology" has drawn the attention of many other disciplines—including experimental philosophy, law, linguistics, psychology, anthropology, the neurosciences and evolutionary biology—bringing a greater awareness of these aspects (Edmonds, 2014). Despite the rather jokey name, we should not be misled: trolleyology is a serious field of inquiry that seeks answers to central questions that invite us to reflect on what we believe is right or wrong and how our preferences and priorities are framed in areas where someone's survival depends on another's death (Kahneman & Tversky, 1984), and again, on how we believe that society can legitimately decide (and communicate) in such delicate circumstances. In zero-sum games—where one player's loss is the other's gain—there can be no mediation between winners and losers, and it is precisely this aspect that makes choice so difficult, especially in cases where there are good reasons to support all options. Trolleyology originates from a number of thought experiments where a runaway trolley is hurtling toward five people tied to the track. If we do nothing, all five will be killed. But if we pull a signal lever and shunt the trolley onto a side track, they will be saved but a single person tied to that track will be killed. These thought experiments, devised to make the ethical issues raised by certain dilemmatic situations easier to grasp and measure, were intended to investigate whether our decisions—hypothetical in this case—tend to hinge more on the consequences of our actions (killing one man to save five) than on their underlying assumptions (that homicide is unacceptable, for example), and what kind of reasoning is deployed in the choices we make when faced with such thorny problems (Edmonds, 2014). The idea is that—even when we ask ourselves abstract questions—we can reflect on what circumstances may be able to change our choices, including those choices that at first blush seemed possible to us: if we say one man should die in order to save five, would we think it equally justifiable for a surgeon to harvest one person's organs, killing him in the process, to transplant them in five other people and save their lives? The ethical experiment thus urges us to think about whether the value we assign to a life can change and, if we judge people's worth by the roles they fill, the responsibilities they have, their age and their abilities, how this variability can change over time for individuals and groups that we feel are less important than others for some reason. As we will see, however, these are not issues that only require us to use our imagination. Often, such dilemmas arise in healthcare systems' everyday practice, unfolding on shaky ground where communication struggles to find the right words and modes of expression. This, then, is all the more reason to take a closer look.

2 Rationing

It is commonly believed that rationing comes to the fore in emergency situations where a sharp rise in the demand for a particular good outstrips its availability and the ability to provide sufficient quantities expeditiously. In reality, the conditions that produce rationing are far more frequent, varied and not always readily recognizable. Budget cuts are an example of a situation where a particular good becomes scarce because of internal policy decisions made as part of healthcare system planning which do not depend on the need to respond to a sudden and, to some extent, unexpected turn of events. Reducing the number of hospital beds or shedding staff, as we said in the first chapter, produces indirect forms of rationing, though it is difficult to gauge their impact on the quality of patient care. How patient wellbeing is linked to the quantity of resources, in fact, is not entirely straightforward:

> Having plenty of staff does not guarantee good care (we saw unacceptable care on well-staffed wards, and excellent care on understaffed ones) but not having enough is a sure path to poor care.
> (Care Quality Commission, 2011, in Klein & Maybin, 2012, p. 39)

For a firmer grip on the question, it may be useful to clarify the meaning of two terms that are often (including in these pages) used almost interchangeably but are not in fact synonymous: *priority-setting* and *rationing*. The first term refers to deciding how to distribute resources among the competing claims of different sectors (healthcare or education, for instance), between different healthcare services or even between different patient groups. Rationing, on the other hand, refers to the effects that allocation decisions have on patients. The fact that resources are allocated to a sector or one of its services—as Klein and Maybin (2012, p. 5) point out—tells us nothing about what this decision will mean for other sectors or the patients in other services. Making a distinction between priority-setting and rationing is important, because it encourages us to look closely at the chain of choices and effects that can take place at various levels, watching the hierarchy of decision-making and the impact that decisions can have as they pass from the highest level (the central government), which distributes resources to the various sectors, to the levels below. At the endpoint of the cascade of decisions, it is up to the clinicians to decide how to allocate their time and resources to patient care in what is known as "bedside rationing". Breaking down the hierarchy of decision-making into its constituent levels makes it possible to determine where action could be taken without throwing the whole burden of responsibility on those who are most exposed to the consequences of the decisions they are forced to make about individual patients. And it is precisely at this level of greatest exposure that tensions are the strongest, and it is here that we must explore what makes decisions publicly acceptable.

To identify the direct and indirect ways of limiting access to resources and care, Klein and Maybin's (2012) study of the UK's National Health Service and how it has changed over the years lists several different forms that rationing can take. In the case of *rationing by denial*, specific types of treatment are excluded from the services on offer, while in other cases—of *rationing by selection*—only certain groups or patients are given treatment. Selection can take place by creating obstacles to accessing resources and treatments that are formally available, for instance, by making it difficult to identify the correct procedures and understand how to obtain the necessary information or find whom to contact—which is known as *rationing by deterrence*—or by shunting patients to other institutions or shuttling them from one service to another, in which case we have *rationing by deflection*. Another less visible but rather pervasive way of limiting access consists of the various forms of *rationing by dilution*, where services are formally available but their quality is reduced, for example, by cuts in staff numbers, in the time devoted to each patient or in the equipment and materials needed for diagnosis and treatment. These dimensions, which as we will see have a number of subdimensions, intersect and combine in ways that depend on circumstances—the 2007 economic crisis, for example, or emergencies like the current pandemic—that are often unpredictable.

We should be aware that dealing with decisions about how resources are allocated does not mean believing that consensus solutions can be found or that any solutions—no matter how carefully crafted—will apply in all places and cases. Why, then, should the issue concern us? And why should we try to find appropriate ways of making these decisions known to the public? One answer could be that we can assume that the consequences of these choices are going to happen anyway, and understanding their underlying logic or seeking to steer them consciously in the desired direction could teach us something (Lupton, 1993). The hope here is that reflexivity and awareness can make it possible—though not certain—for us to become more effective at clarifying the implications of these choices and pave the way to new and perhaps better, albeit always perfectible, collective answers. Certainties are few, as Klein & Malbin remind us, but the questions we must ask ourselves abound, and none are easy to answer. For example, the two scholars ask: "Should rationing be explicit or implicit? Is the way decisions are taken as important as—perhaps even more important than—the criteria and methodology used?" (2012, p. 2).

Despite the many uncertainties that must inevitably be acknowledged, a broader-based attention to the dimensions of problem-setting seems to be very much a part of the process of improving problem-solving capabilities. Accordingly, in the following pages, we will dig down into the reasons that make it difficult to deal publicly with rationing issues, starting with a short review of their often contradictory facets and then outlining a few of the strategies that practice and research have used to tackle the field's many complications.

3 Areas that "do not stand the light of day"

The thought experiments and Oregon's healthcare policies are not central to the line of thought we will propose here. Nevertheless, they help us bring two important points into sharper focus: the first has to do with the nature of the questions facing us, which often makes us forget that the problems of allocating resources and rationing have a lengthy history in healthcare system practices as well as in choice theory and thus do not arise only in emergencies such as the 2020 pandemic.

The second point is that issues of justice and fairness—and, especially, how they translate into practice—inhabit an objectively complex sphere, where the forms of communication are of paramount importance. The questions here are not limited to who should make the decisions but also concern whether (and how) decisions should be explicit, or in other words discussed and justified to the public. The dilemmas that questions involve are likely to lead to strategies of denial and repression and make it difficult to explain the assumptions behind choices, given that they could involve visions that are potentially irreconcilable and thus risky for those who, like the institutions, need to have the legitimacy of their decisions acknowledged at all times. As a result, particularly complex policy issues often tend to be removed from the public debate because they are highly divisive, or are presented in terms of partisan politics even though their actual content might have some appeal across party divisions:

> Politicians are obviously concerned with the impact that policies could have on society (or rather, on certain social categories), but what concerns them most is the impact of policies on politics and its equilibriums.
>
> (Bobbio et al., 2015, p. 520)

While the problem of how to allocate scarce resources and communicate choices is central to both politics and the economy and is thus not new, the particular nature of the goods we are dealing with here—whose value goes beyond merely financial considerations—poses a number of specific problems. What Kahn-Harris calls "denialism"—denying truths that have been shown to be grounded in fact—can have dramatic consequences. While denial chiefly takes the form of repression (Cohen, 2001), denialism, by shaping narratives that refuse to recognize that a problem exists, not only shifts attention elsewhere but also confuses causes and responsibilities and makes it impossible to provide the resources needed to address the problem, as in the following example:

> In South Africa, President Thabo Mbeki, in office between 1999 and 2008, was influenced by AIDS denialists, who deny the link between HIV and AIDS (or even HIV's existence) and cast doubt on the effectiveness of anti-retrovirals. His reluctance to implement national treatment programmes that made use of anti-retrovirals has been estimated to have cost the lives of 330,000 people.
>
> (Kahn-Harris, 2018, p. 4)

As in the case of denial, we are not dealing here with exclusively psychological mechanisms but with a complex and changeable mixture of ignorance, unawareness, special interests and an often instrumental use or concealment of information. Though the consequences of denialism, which can be seen in the responses of a number of world leaders to the Covid-19 pandemic, would deserve a study of their own, we will limit ourselves here to citing them as an example of the complex ties between communication and the allocation mechanisms employed by those who have the power to choose.

Whether they are denied or openly addressed, allocation decisions are often complicated and painful, especially for those on the receiving end. Not surprisingly, Calabresi & Bobbit employed the expression "tragic choices" a few decades ago to denote decisions that—in extreme cases—can be matters of life and death (1978) and thus entail an enormous involvement, emotional and otherwise, on the part of actors caught up in circumstances of considerable ambiguity. To illustrate some of the reasons that make it easier to remove these choices from the public debate and present a few of the strategies that have been concretely adopted to encourage discussion and agreement about intrinsically divisive issues, the following pages will review the ambiguities involved in selecting the criteria for resource allocation together with some of the implications that follow from these choices.

4 The heterogeneity of principles

Scholarly attention to the heterogeneity of moral principles gained impetus in the 1940s, when subjectivism's claim that there are no objective moral truths clashed with logical positivism's defense of their importance (Edmonds, 2014). In the following decades, starting with Rawls' work (1971)—which sought to develop a conception of distributive justice that could go beyond the utilitarian principles that he believed to be detrimental to minorities—a sizable body of studies began to take a closer look at healthcare, training their sights specifically on the theoretical aspects and the repercussions of putting theory into practice (see, for example, Ham & Pickard, 1998; Cookson & Dolan, 2000; Jones et al., 2004; Berney et al., 2005).

At the beginning of the 1990s, Elster enumerated several principles[3]—applicable not only to healthcare—whereby institutions can establish priorities for allocating scarce resources and then turns to the dilemmas that can arise when these principles are applied. Following Elster's terminology, allocative issues can be classified according to whether or not goods are scarce and indivisible. In certain instances, scarcity is induced by emergencies, as is the case of the shortage of intensive care beds or ventilators during the Covid-19 pandemic, while in others it results from other kinds of problem rather than a lack of the good itself: cost, for example, can prevent everyone who needs a good from being able to have it. As for indivisibility, a cycle of treatment or a hospital bed is a good that cannot be divided among several patients, which makes dealing with allocative problems particularly complicated. The difficulty in agreeing on principles is—as we have said—a source of conflicts and friction, given that the actors involved may have entirely irreconcilable points of view. Even if an agreement is reached or a decision is able to gain headway, not all of the properties on which the different principles are based can be readily observed. Though in some cases they rest on objective and/or measurable criteria (age, for example), in others they "cannot be ascertained without some discretionary assessment", and it is thus much harder to find ways to justify their adoption in the public's eyes, given that it is more likely that they will be considered arbitrary or self-serving (Elster, 1992, p. 69).

The problem, as we will see, is that none of these principles is self-evident or necessarily compelling. We can distinguish, for example, between principles that refer to the properties of the potential beneficiaries and those that focus on the potential benefits to the community, but each of these sets of principles runs through a virtually infinite gamut of distinctions that makes it difficult to find our bearings or take up a stance of any kind. We will now take a look at some of these distinctions.

Say that in order to decide who will receive a certain resource, we concentrate on the properties of the potential beneficiaries. In this case, one possibility is to consider elements defined by status or in other words "principles based on observable biophysical properties or on social and legal features that are a matter of public record" (Elster, 1992, p. 76). These features include age, gender, religion and ethnic, civil, family, residential or occupational status, as well as physical features such as height or other attributes such as literacy. Even if we limit ourselves to properties of this kind, it is not easy to set priorities for allocating a given good, and plausible arguments can be advanced for diametrically opposed decisions. As regards age, we could argue that the elderly deserve a particular treatment by virtue of their past contributions to society, for example, because of lengthy employment in socially useful or stressful jobs, or because they have a specific kind of experience. On the other hand, we could also think in terms of efficiency in using the resource in question, giving the elderly less priority than young people "partly because treatment is less likely to succeed, given the medical problems correlated with age, and partly because even if it does work the old have fewer years left to live" (Elster, 1992, p. 77). If we decide to allocate resources to the young, it is then necessary to specify who counts as young and, for example, whether we believe that priority should go to children or to young adults who already have roles and positions of responsibility in society. Nor can we expect automatic agreement on the age to be used as the cut-off point, or on what to do with people who are just below this threshold. It should be clear now that there is no single, correct answer and that the various approaches depend to a large extent on the conceptions of justice we choose, on whether or not there are rules, norms and customs, on cultural background and on the role, interests and preferences of those who are called upon to choose.

If we decide to base our principles on other conditions rather than the properties of the individual, the problems seem even greater. Elster distinguishes between need, interpreted on the basis of the individual level of welfare that precedes—for example—taking a scarce drug, and a criterion that considers the possible increment of welfare that this drug could produce. This is a problem we encountered in the second chapter with the story of Annapurna. Here again, it might seem equally plausible to provide a particular treatment to those whose condition is worse or to those who could benefit most even if their original condition was not particularly critical. Need and level of wellbeing are thus not objective or measurable criteria, as they necessarily bring discretionary assessments into play which are not easy to agree on or communicate publicly. Deciding whether to base allocative decisions on the greater capacity to benefit or on the rule of rescue—i.e., providing resources to whoever is in worse condition, cost what it may—means choosing between two criteria that are both legitimate but can come into conflict. But the complications do not end here. There is yet another criterion, one which hinges—often implicitly—on a judgment about the individuals to whom the resource is to be provided.

4.1 Who is deserving and who is not?

Alongside assessments of individuals' greater or lesser capacity to respond well to treatment, other judgments may creep in, which place people along a hierarchy of value on the basis of certain properties, such as age, their state of health or their presumed responsibility for their own condition. Consequently, it may be that access to scarce resources does not depend exclusively on the capacity to benefit from them but will also reflect the greater value which is assigned to some people and denied to others. Deciding whether or not someone deserves to receive a treatment or win access to a medication that is not available to everyone brings together many aspects that entail controversial assessments. Deserving and undeserving, worthy and unworthy are labels—rather than self-evident categories—that once attached will invariably bring significant consequences. It is a distinction that tends to be associated with individual behaviors and draws a line between those who are not believed to have taken enough responsibility for maintaining their own health and thus can to some extent be blamed for their condition, and those whose health has suffered because of circumstances beyond their control. In the first case, as is sometimes argued, the community has no obligation to earmark collective resources to those who were the first to neglect their health. But is it really possible to discriminate so sharply between deserving and undeserving, in a way that everyone would agree with? Can people who have a substance abuse problem or an eating disorder be held responsible for their problems and thus be considered unworthy of accessing treatment for other diseases they might develop? Once again, there is no easy answer. It must be borne in mind that these problems could stem from pathological conditions that have nothing to do with what the individual may or may not want, and that people who have them could have experienced circumstances in which they were the victim: they may have been abused, for example, or been involved in other complex situations that triggered inappropriate coping responses for which they can hardly be blamed. But if the person in question is considered responsible for their own condition, would the idea of denying treatment seem acceptable to us? Or would it seem acceptable only if there were not enough resources to go around? As can be seen, in the distinction between deserving and undeserving, cultural conceptions and ideas of value are prone to short-circuit, preventing us from clearly and unquestionably identifying which lives are valuable and ought thus to be saved in preference to others.

As Clavien & Hurst argue, in order to make a distinction between deserving and undeserving patients, it would at least be necessary to be able to identify "the minimal conditions for 'practical' and for 'moral' responsibility attribution" (2019, p. 175). While certain individual behaviors or lifestyles can increase the risk of developing a certain disease, the possible increase is associated by definition with a probability which does not mean that the illness will materialize. Illness, in fact, is always the outcome of multiple causal factors, including genetic predisposition, environmental background and even happenstance or bad luck. This wide range of causal factors also applies to those who lead unhealthy lifestyles or whose behavior can increase the likelihood of falling ill. Consequently, deserving and undeserving cannot be reduced to a black and white distinction but is a matter of degree: the effect of specific circumstances that are not necessarily stable but can change over time. The distinction inevitably entails value judgments about individual conditions, and it is clear that if healthcare providers whose profession exposes them to greater risks than the rest of the population fall ill, no one would consider them to be blameworthy.

Given these premises, Clavien & Hurst maintain that responsibility cannot be attributed automatically, as it is necessary to identify the specific circumstances that each individual must face and the factors that could have reduced responsibility, independently of the choices the individual made. If we believe that this distinction is meaningful, we must, at the very least, check whether the individual in question had the opportunity—and was aware of having it—to make other choices. For example, no one could blame patients for not taking a drug if they could not afford it. More generally, it is necessary that people be informed of the alternatives open to them, that they have the time to think over their options, and that they be able to grasp the implications of their actions. As we mentioned earlier, individuals' opportunities and hence the responsibility that can be attributed to them can also be limited by specific circumstances: being of low socioeconomic status, for example, or suffering from mental disorders or other conditions that can impair their cognitive capacities and cloud their understanding.

It might seem obvious that if I have mental problems I should not be held responsible (or at least not entirely) for my behavior. Many countries' legal systems, for example, excuse mentally incompetent defendants from full criminal liability. In point of fact, however, we must stress that none of this is all that obvious, as can be seen from the persistent stigma—in the public discourse and in the healthcare system itself[4]—that attaches to conditions that do not depend on individual behaviors, like mental illness (Knaak et al., 2017) or dementia (Batsch et al., 2012). The stigma is even greater in the case of conditions that are considered—rightly or wrongly[5]—to have a more direct link with individual choices (Marroni et al., 2018; Brown, 2019).

The point is that the stigma—whatever its origins—associated with certain conditions has major consequences for patients and their families and severely curtails their ability to receive adequate support from care providers or even from the communities they live in.

These reflections about whether patients are deserving or undeserving and their responsibility for their own illness point to the need for greater attention to the concept of responsibility: not only that of the patients, but that of their care providers and the healthcare system as a whole, which is tasked with determining the best ways of supporting those in need, whatever the circumstances that caused their condition. This—as Coulehan and colleagues argue—calls for going beyond the "myopic model of dyadic relationships" between patient and physicians and moving toward a social conception of responsibility which, like Engel's biopsychosocial model (1977), takes a broader view of illness, its determinants and the strategies for dealing with it:

> To understand patient's illnesses, we need to appreciate the economic, social, and cultural context in which they arise. Likewise, to treat them effectively, we often need to design and implement social intervention.
>
> (Coulehan et al., 2003, p. 26)

Assigning responsibility by means of judgments about worthiness and unworthiness is thus a delicate operation that requires attention to the various macro and microlevels involved in healthcare practice. For that reason, careful thought must be given to the principles used and to the representations and discourses that circulate more or less intentionally in society. If this broader view is not taken, the repercussions risk penalizing those who are already most fragile:

> By taking the task of reflecting seriously on objective criteria for responsibility attribution, we have shown that patients with unhealthy lifestyles are often disproportionately held responsible and sanctioned for their health conditions. In the light of our analysis, the rhetoric of patients' responsibility turns out to be an illegitimate and hypocritical opportunity to punish those who have behavioral habits that are condemned socially.
>
> (Clavien & Hurst, 2019, p. 14)

Despite the complications we have outlined, even using criteria that are decoupled from individual characteristics to decide who will receive resources that are not sufficient for everyone does not make the choice any easier. For example, egalitarian principles that adopt a criterion of absolute equality by dividing a scarce good into equal shares or which give everyone the same chance of access do not necessarily result in a fairer situation, given that each person needs a specific quantity of the good in question in order to benefit from it, and receiving more of it would be a waste while receiving less would make it useless. Likewise, the use of lotteries or rotation procedures to determine who receives the good is not applicable in certain cases (access to prescription drugs, for example) but useful in others, such as preventing corruption in the selection of jurors or politicians, where random selection could have undeniable advantages (Elster, 1992, p. 72). Time-related principles are another example. Here, scarce goods are allocated on the basis of a particular time associated with them, such as the appearance of a disease's first symptoms or the moment a patient is put on a waiting list for an organ transplant. According to Elster, these criteria can contribute to simplifying the decision in some circumstances:

> With some medical goods, time spent on the waiting list is a proxy for medical need, since a patient's condition often deteriorates over time. A list, like a queue, is a self-sorting device that does not require controversial and costly discretionary decisions.
>
> (Elster, 1992, p. 74)

However, this simplification may be only apparent in settings with high levels of corruption, where there could be legitimate doubts about whether the principle in question has been correctly translated into practice. In addition, for any given time spent on a waiting list, it would still be necessary to apply further criteria, with all the problems mentioned above.

5 The heterogeneity of the actors

Having so many principles is not the only source of complication. Yet another has to do with the fact that they must be selected and agreed on by an equally heterogeneous set of actors who have a say in allocation decisions or are affected by them. Elster distinguishes between first-, second- and third-order actors, referring respectively to the political authorities, the institutions whose job is to handle allocation situations in practice and the recipients of the allocated good. In addition, these three sets could also be influenced by public opinion, which has significant power in legitimatizing choices because of its ability to call the choosers into question. Each of the actors decides whether criteria are desirable on the basis of their own specific motivations. For example, the political actors and local institutions may be chiefly interested in efficiency, with the risk of causing additional distortions:

> Being under relentless pressure from innumerable interest groups as well as administrative agencies, they will be reluctant to allocate funds for a particular scarce good unless they can be confident that the funds will be efficiently used.
>
> (1992, p. 180)

These actors may also feel that equity matters, if for no other reason than because politicians and institutions fear scandals and are thus constantly concerned with deferring to public opinion which sees equity as paramount. The third-order actors, or in other words those who have direct personal experience of a certain condition, are chiefly moved by self-interest, even though—as in the case of the first- and second-order actors—here too there may be broader arguments that appeal to considerations of equity and efficiency.

It should also be borne in mind that referring to the point of view and perspectives of the different actors in no way implies that each holds a single conception that is not in turn roiled with divisions and conflicts about the criteria or methods for making concrete decisions to act. The fact that many different actors are involved thus gives rise to a new set of problems regarding how their preferences try, and are at times able, to aggregate in order to yield what in the end will become the final allocative scheme. The complexity of the mechanisms behind coalition building and bargaining, particularly in view of the different amount of power held by the actors and institutional levels, can cause the choices to diverge significantly from the basic principles that each participant originally intended to espouse, introducing further complications when attempts are made after the fact to reconstruct the rationale and produce consistent narratives. The instability of preferences is thus linked both to the variability of coalitions and bargains and to the fact that no choice will be able to make everyone happy:

> Because any scheme will create objections in some quarters, and because the faults of the system in place tend to be more vivid than the flaws of the alternatives, we often observe unstable oscillations and perpetual modifications.
>
> (Elster, 1992, p. 137)

The difficulty in defining principles and justifying the resulting practices publicly makes it extremely risky for politicians and institutions to reveal what is going on and bring it into the public debate: "Because tragic choices do not stand the light of day, they cannot be made by principle conforming to the *condition of publicity* that constrains allocation in democratic societies" (Elster, 1992, p. 9).

And this is the paradox that inevitably accompanies such choices: they must be discussed, but at the same time it is necessary to avoid debate on issues that are all too likely to set tempers aflame, widen rifts and erode the legitimacy of the institutions involved. Forty years ago, Calabresi and Bobbit (1978) already felt that the situation was so complex as to leave little room for hope. Their assessment was pessimistic in the main, as they held that, essentially, society could do little more than make the best of a bad job, trying to downplay the fact that some people are inevitably chosen to live and others to die.

5.1 From theory to practice: the role of healthcare providers

As we have seen, having to choose on the basis of abstract principles is one thing, and having to decide—as physicians do—in emergency situations involving real, flesh and blood patients whose suffering must be alleviated is another thing altogether. These are central aspects that deserve more of our time. However, earmarking resources for those who are worst off and need urgent help is often not the same as maximizing the general welfare and does not result in an optimal allocation of available goods. Elster tells us of a California hospital where "the shift from the 'most critical' to the 'most salvageable' standard in the allocation of intensive care ward space" reduced the mortality rate from 80% to 20% (1992, pp. 86–87). While this figure is significant in terms of overall efficiency and the number of lives saved, physicians frequently resist adopting this second standard even though it brings an improvement in the general wellbeing. There can be several reasons for this. For example, physicians tend to act—and are trained to do so—in emergency conditions and on the basis of immediate need, while they are less inclined to take an approach that considers what the end result might be in aggregate terms of total welfare. A number of factors, including the so-called *norm of compassion*, contribute to encouraging physician responses that are more oriented toward the patient than to the efficient use of scarce goods. "The principle of channeling medical resources toward the critically ill patients, even when they would do more good in others" appears to be linked, not only to empathy with the suffering, but also to the *certainty effect* that leads physicians to be swayed more by the "clear and present danger" incurred by critically ill patients than by the "more uncertain and conjectural" risks faced by patients in less serious condition (Elster, 1992, p. 147).

The time that physicians devote to patients—which the latter regard as a central factor in evaluating the quality of care—appears to have decreasing marginal utility, even though physicians seem to apply a *norm of thoroughness*:

> This implies that if the doctor makes a very thorough examination of the patient, his behavior is not instrumentally rational with respect to the objective of saving life or improving health. Other patients might benefit much more from the time he spends on the last and most esoteric tests. Nevertheless, doctors seem to follow a norm of thoroughness, which tells them that once a patient has been admitted, he or she should get "the full treatment".
>
> (Elster, 1992, p. 148)

These few remarks can give some idea of how central physicians are to decision-making and how difficult it is to expect care providers to adopt and apply businesslike standards (for budget savings, for example) that are far removed from their values and anything they have been trained to do. Once again, it is clear that which allocative principles are chosen is heavily dependent on the role one occupies, the rules that apply in the particular context and the way this context affects how the actors' competences change over time.

6 Models of choice and public discussion processes

According to the *Accountability for Reasonableness Framework* (Daniels & Sabin, 2002, in Klein & Maybin, 2012, p. 9), the criteria to be considered in making decisions should include publicity, relevance, challenge and revision, and regulation. This means that allocation decisions should be public, based on reasons that fair-minded people would agree are relevant and not made once and for all but open to challenge and revision. Lastly, the decision-making process should be subject to forms of public regulation to ensure that the other criteria are applied. But however reasonable general principles may be in theory, translating them into practice is never free from problems. Though there is unanimous consent that decisions about priorities should be public, how to proceed is not equally clear. Should the reasonableness of choices be justified after the fact, for instance, by clarifying the circumstances in which they were made? Or should the parties who could be affected be involved in the discussions preceding the choice? If so, who exactly should be involved: the patients or representatives of the public? Not everyone believes that engaging the public directly in rationing decisions is useful, and several studies have found that the majority of the public feels that these choices should be left to physicians, inasmuch as they are experts and thus have a better understanding of their implications and repercussions in clinical practice (Chisholm et al., 2009).

On the other hand, the difficulty in agreeing on values and how to translate them into healthcare practices, as well as the awareness that experts' stances can also be controversial and "medical opinion can speak with many voices" (Klein & Maybin, 2012, p. 8), have led to many attempts over the years to find the most appropriate ways to legitimize choices and understand who ought to make them. As we saw in the second chapter, public choices are a complex area involving many different perspectives. As regards allocation decisions in particular, one of the first distinctions we can make is between models that propose to develop some sort of mechanism using the data collected about the advantages of each option and those based on engaging a set of stakeholders and shareholders in some form of deliberative participation.

One example of the first approach is the so-called *Technocratic Model*. This model is based on the idea that making choices should be as free as possible from subjective assessments and judgments. Decisions are thus entrusted to expert panels that rely on the available empirical evidence about the effectiveness of new drugs, for example, or the comparative benefits to patients of different treatments. To decide who should receive a particular treatment, for instance, the potential beneficiaries' conditions are compared using the *Quality Adjusted Life Year* (QALY), a unit of measure consisting of two dimensions:

> The first is the length of life—months or years—that the patient can expect following treatment. The second is the quality of that life. The quality is measured on a scale ranging from 0 (death) to 1 (perfect health). The scale takes into account mobility, pain or discomfort, anxiety or depression and the ability to pursue the usual activities of daily living.
>
> (Klein & Maybin, 2012, p. 11)

The model is interesting because it seeks to relieve individual healthcare providers of the burden of choice through a procedure which hopes to be objective. Calculating the QALY of a standard treatment and that of a new treatment makes it possible—according to the approach's supporters—to compare the cost of the treatment which is most advantageous for the patient and at the same time to assess its sustainability for the National Health Service as compared to standard care. Once the cost-effectiveness of the new treatment has been established, it is still necessary to set the thresholds for acceptable spending. But since there are no objective criteria for deciding when a cost increase can be considered acceptable and what level of expenditure each service can (or intends) to incur, the model has drawn extensive criticism centering on the fact that at a certain point it is still necessary to make the value judgment that the model set out to avoid. Critics have also questioned whether fair choices can be made if cost-effectiveness takes priority in allocating resources. Indeed, QALYs can also be used to decide who will receive a resource which is not available for everyone. Here the problem lies in the fact that in calculating the benefit that two patients could receive from a particular treatment—even assuming the same life expectancy for both after treatment—if one of the two were disabled, his or her QALY score would in any case be lower than the other's. With an assessment that prioritizes the cost–benefit ratio, whoever has no additional problems will thus always receive the resource in question, which clearly runs counter to ethical principles and to laws barring disability-based discrimination in access to care.[6]

A second group of models starts from very different assumptions: rather than using automatic mechanisms to make allocative decisions, a central role is assigned to processes of public discussion and deliberation to establish what aspects should be prioritized at a given time and in a given context. Here again, this is a large set of models and practices that in recent decades have enjoyed considerable currency in Italy and elsewhere (Bohman, 1998; Regonini, 2005; Pellizzoni, 2007). As Bobbio points out, the umbrella term deliberative processes covers a disparate array of theoretical approaches and practical implementations that share

> a common wager, viz., that making public choices can benefit from the discursive and informed interaction between citizens who have different (or opposing) opinions or interests.
>
> (2013, p. 12)

A few words are in order concerning these processes because, as we will see, even if the goals of these forms of citizen participation are only partially achieved in practice, deliberative exchanges between the actors (Niemeyer & Dryzek, 2007) can yield the positive repercussions of what Abbott (2003, pp. 120–134) calls "argument heuristics", which are ways of turning familiar arguments into something new by problematizing the obvious, reversing assumptions and turning them on their head, or reconceptualizing what would be possible if we look at a problem from a different, and perhaps unusual, perspective. Here again, however, not all of the problems are solved, and deliberative practices can also be put to instrumental use to give the impression that public input is considered important but in fact reasserting decisions that have already been made (Regonini, 2005).

Precisely because of the difficulties of understanding beforehand what can be achieved through stakeholder participation, the literature on deliberative processes acknowledges that the value of discussing issues of collective interest is largely procedural, as it is a by-product of the dynamics established by the participants which helps information to circulate more effectively and makes it less likely to be manipulated by those who hold more power; in addition, it can encourage the parties to admit their own errors and cognitive short-circuits. According to Bobbio (2013), though there are procedural advantages to be gained from deliberative processes, we should also question the effects of the substantive advantages, or in other words the extent to which these processes can in practice make it possible to arrive at consensus-based criteria and solutions. We should thus ask where their quality lies and whether agreement can actually be reached through these methods of engagement. There are in fact many aspects that make further thought necessary in order to understand if and how these approaches can help participants find more areas of common ground and lead to better-informed choices. These are important questions, in view of the high costs—economic and otherwise—of participative methods.

Bobbio reminds us that the participants' preferences are not necessarily extraneous to the deliberative process and can thus be redefined and brought into sharper focus in the course of the discussions. However, he also emphasizes that even though these preferences may change, it is not clear how they can be brought together at the implementation stage or how previously unconsidered aspects that emerge during the discussion can be taken into account.

6.1 A few suggestions about the use of deliberative practices in healthcare

A variety of studies have investigated these principles' journey from theory to practice. Sabik and Lie (2008), for example, analyzed the criteria used to set priorities for allocating healthcare resources in eight countries. Their goal was to evaluate how consistent the processes for selecting allocative criteria were with their subsequent application, hoping that the analysis could provide lessons from the countries' experience despite the differences in their healthcare systems. The countries were divided into two groups on the basis of how abstract their priority setting approaches are: the first group—which includes Norway, the Netherlands, Sweden and Denmark—used approaches that are more centered on outlining general principles such as human dignity or need and solidarity, while the second—consisting of Israel, New Zealand, the US state of Oregon and the United Kingdom—focused on establishing the circumstances in which the net gain to society is higher than the costs incurred or whether costly health treatments made possible by new technologies are justifiable and sustainable, and, if so, on what basis.

It is interesting to note that despite the differences in their healthcare systems, all eight countries took identifying the broadest possible selection methods very seriously and sought to promote public input and discussion about priority setting. Starting in the 1980s, all the countries thus set up government commissions consisting of healthcare experts and, in some countries, government officials and representatives of patients' associations. Sabik & Lie report widespread difficulties in producing robust results and note that, despite the enormous outlay of effort and resources, the principles outlined by the commissions had little direct impact on their countries' healthcare policies because of their abstractness or the difficulties in translating them into practice. Disappointingly, this would also appear to apply to the countries that took a more pragmatic approach. In general, attempts at public involvement and participation, for example, through patients' associations, seem to have had some effect only at the initial stages of the process, at most leading to a greater degree of acceptance of the adopted criteria but not to their revision. On the basis of these findings, the study explicitly recommends expert-led processes because of the limited feasibility of extensive public involvement (Sabik & Lie, 2008).

Though as we have seen, participative approaches are beset by problems in establishing discussion and choosing the interlocutors and methods to be used, they have attracted increasing attention over the years, especially as regards their implementation when unexpected circumstances arise (Koonin et al., 2020; Emanuel et al., 2020). For example, the field of Disaster Medicine[7] has explored how tools can be identified which can be deployed before emergencies occur, thus helping those who may be called upon to deal with difficult allocation decisions like those involving insufficient quantities of life-sustaining resources (Waeckerle et al., 1994). In particular, a study by Biddison et al. (2018, 2019) sought to extend community engagement in the tragic choices discussed earlier to include the general public as well as healthcare and disaster professionals and encourage broad participation. The objective was to investigate the public's opinions and values regarding how scarce mechanical ventilators should be allocated during an influenza pandemic, with the ultimate goal of developing an allocation framework that could be applied in a health emergency, when decisions must be made on the fly, and in-depth deliberations are not feasible.

Conducted in Maryland between 2012 and 2014, the mixed-method community engagement study held at least one forum for laypersons and one for healthcare and disaster workers in each of the state's five emergency management regions. A few words are in order concerning the approach, both to outline its details and illustrate the complexity of the practices employed to ensure that the study's results would be as robust as possible and to encourage reflection about why the outcomes of deliberative processes frequently fail to be reflected in institutional practice.

The study included a quantitative evaluation that developed a scoring system used to determine priority in accessing resources. Priority was given to patients who were assigned the lowest total scores in triage assessment. The scoring system primarily took into account the likelihood of short-term and long-term survival, with scores rising for patients with comorbid conditions and as patient age increased. Other conditions considered included pregnancy: pregnant patients were given a 1-point reduction on their priority score if the fetus was healthy, and it was thus reasonably likely that the child's life could be saved in addition to that of the mother. Where patients had the same priority score after applying these criteria, the model envisaged that ventilators should be allocated on a first-come, first-served basis or through some form of lottery. In addition, the model provided several exclusion criteria, i.e., conditions that would in any case reduce patients' chances of survival and thus made them ineligible to receive resources. These conditions included cardiac arrest, severe burns over 50% of the total body surface and advanced and irreversible neurologic events or conditions.

In a pandemic, moreover, patients presenting with respiratory failure resulting from the pandemic disease and those needing a ventilator for another reason were scored on the same scale and thus had the same chances of access to life-sustaining treatment. Lastly, the model required that patients in critical condition be stabilized and given temporary support while awaiting triage.

In addition to the scoring system, the study carried out a qualitative analysis to identify the major themes to be addressed and to characterize the community values regarding allocation decisions. Given the variety of considerations on which published recommendations for allocating life-support measures during a public health emergency are based, the researchers believed that the discussion should also include the public, who will bear the consequences of allocation decisions. The objective was not so much to reach a consensus, as to gain a wider knowledge of community perspectives and values so that what happens during a crisis can be understood and accepted by the general public. In contrast with much of the literature, the objective here was not to present recommendations offered by panels of experts but to explore the views of those who might find themselves on the frontline in emergency situations, as patients or healthcare professionals.

Study procedures were pilot-tested in two distinct communities, viz., one inner city and one suburban setting. The findings of these pilot sessions were then used to revise and specify the form and content of the subsequent stages. The support materials to be shared with forum participants to elicit their informed opinion were selected by a multidisciplinary team consisting of experts in critical care and emergency medicine, emergency management, bioethics, social science and democratic deliberation theory and methods. The team also developed two surveys that were administered to participants before and after the forum. According to the study protocol, each forum started with an orientation period in which the information contained in a background document distributed to the participants in advance was reviewed, and the schedule for the following stages was presented. The participants, who were divided into small groups ensuring racial and ethnic diversity, were asked to discuss the following questions: "What should we do in situations in which there are more patients needing ventilators than there are ventilators to use?" and "Should health-care providers ever be allowed to remove a ventilator from one patient who needs it to survive and give it to another who also needs it to survive?" Forums were conducted by trained facilitators who led the discussion about the ethical principles that participants might use alone or in combination to establish priorities in cases where there were not enough resources to go around. Participants could also indicate other principles or factors affecting their views. The ethical principles discussed in forums concern prioritizing those most likely to survive the current illness; those most likely to live the longest after recovery (considering comorbid conditions); those who have lived fewer life stages; those who have particular instrumental value to others in a pandemic or principles such as "first come, first served" or lottery (Biddison et al., 2018, p. 189).

The study also collected data from exit interviews with a subset of participants who were asked to provide feedback concerning their opinion of the forum process and their understanding of the issues that were discussed. The interviewees voiced a number of concerns that are unlikely to be brought into focus when discussing principles in the abstract (the trolleyology we spoke of at the beginning of the chapter), including fears not only about the choices but about how their repercussions will be handled and the resulting need to provide patients who cannot be given ventilators with some form of support to make their condition more "comfortable" as death approaches. A significant number of concerns—expressed by laypeople and frontline clinicians alike—involved the fear that it would be difficult to ensure conditions that respect the dignity of all patients—those that make it through the illness as well as those who do not—as well as worries that inequities (between the insured and uninsured, and those affecting certain perceived "undesirable" groups such as undocumented immigrants, prisoners or drug addicts) could be replicated and thus stressed the need for greater caution in applying criteria that distinguish between the deserving and the undeserving.

On the whole, deliberation—though complex, costly and time-consuming for the researchers as well as the participants—was found to be useful in drawing attention to the lessons learned from the experience and in reflecting on how better tools can be developed which take the legitimate concerns voiced by laypeople and care providers into account.

First, it was noted that if a deliberative arena is to be able to explore the possible implications and dilemmas that complex issues could entail, it not only must be carefully organized with a clear definition of who does what, but should also be led by trained facilitators who can act as effective go-betweens in creating an open environment. Discussing the criteria for allocating ventilators, moreover, brought the ambivalence that inevitably accompanies difficult decisions out into the open. One aspect that thus became evident was the unresolvable contradiction posed by the fact that the difficulty of involving a broader public in discussion principles is at the same time the condition that makes it possible to enrich the debate so that different perspectives emerge and interact. This is important because, by recognizing that there is no one best solution, no one best approach, it helps relieve tensions if the process fails to meet expectations. It is also interesting to note that some of the issues brought up in the forums did not figure in the recommendations and guidelines that were the starting point for the study. In particular, the values of the lay participants and frontline clinicians sometimes diverged from expert guidance. As Biddison and colleagues emphasize, this is an important finding that should inform policy-making and communication:

> Although formal guidance has espoused principles such as fairness in the abstract, many participants expressed their understanding of those principles

in more concrete experiential terms, including fears that allocation decisions will follow locally known patterns of inequity/unfairness. The finding of local ethical "dialects", suggests the potential need for policy makers to communicate the rationale for an allocation framework in terms that are salient for specific audiences.

(Biddison et al., 2018, p. 194)

Alongside the lessons learned from the deliberative process, Biddison and colleagues acknowledge a number of limitations to the study that speak to the inherent complexity of any attempt to develop tools that can yield generalizable findings: for example, the time commitment required of participants may have introduced nonparticipation bias, while the sample may not have been fully representative of the diversity of the general population, an aspect which is all the more relevant in contexts such as the United States, where ethnicity weighs significantly on access to healthcare resources.

Although the allocation framework has not been formally adopted in Maryland's preparedness plans, some of the considerations that emerged during its development provide insights that can be applied to our understanding of the Covid-19 pandemic. Most centrally, the framework demonstrated the weight that transparency and public awareness have in securing the cooperation of communities faced with extreme conditions. We may legitimately ask whether the reactions shown during the pandemic by a portion of the population in many countries—anger, denial and refusal to act cautiously and follow the institutions' advice as businesses gradually reopened—could have been moderated if more attention had been given to ensuring that information circulated effectively or to forms of public discussion before the emergency struck. When widespread instinctive reactions are accompanied by denial or denialism, strategies designed to promote a better understanding of what is going on or provide support for care providers which include opportunities for public discussion and input seem to improve the ability to deal with uncertainty and field more targeted responses to protect individual and collective health. During dramatic events, participatory planning, coordination and communication seem to make it possible—not, perhaps, to vanquish uncertainty—but to at least agree on how to manage it without undermining the credibility of the processes and institutions involved.

Though the deliberative experiments we have described were far from finding the key to solving resource allocation and priority-setting problems, these experiences demonstrate that it is essential to make efforts to manage uncertainty and find processes which show that choices are legitimate and can help make them publicly acceptable. This means focusing on all the many steps that can strengthen the legitimacy of decisions, even when they can been seen to have limits: in addition to considering the criteria that can have an impact on how fair the resource allocation process is, it is crucial to ask ourselves how the decisions are perceived by public opinion, the amount of trust placed in the decision-makers and the procedures whereby the public is concretely involved in arriving at decisions and discussing their outcomes.

After these reflections on public involvement in decisions, we will now turn to how a different kind of information circulated during the pandemic months. How much space did the media give to the dilemmas we discussed in the preceding pages? And more generally, what kind of relationship forms between the media and health in the midst of emergencies?

7 Images and representations of healthcare from the Covid-19 pandemic[8]

The Covid-19 pandemic thrust us suddenly into a universe where the problems and thought experiments associated with "trolleyology" became unexpectedly and alarmingly concrete, in very dramatic ways (Lusardi & Tomelleri, 2020). It is interesting to note that—at least in Italy—the public debate that took shape in the major national newspapers showed almost no trace of the complexity of tragic choices that we spoke of earlier. By contrast, there was an immediate flurry of attention in medical and epidemiological circles and in the social sciences, producing a sizable body of work that grew with incredible speed.

Between February and July 2020, representations of the National Health Service in Italy's largest dailies concentrated chiefly on whether it could hold up under the strain, noting that the service's long-standing problems complicated its ability to cope with the pandemic. For example, the papers dwelt on how continual budget cuts had contributed to the shortage of intensive care beds during the emergency, and in fact, given the lack of resources, the regional health services were absolved of the need to adopt and implement the "National Pandemic Influenza Preparedness Plan", which had last been updated in 2010. The fact that a large proportion of deaths took place in care homes for the elderly then shifted the debate to the scant consideration given to older people even in a highly familistic culture such as Italy's, and how this led the pandemic's extent and risks to be underestimated until it became clear that the country's senior citizens were the hardest hit (Arlotti & Ranci, 2020). Thus, of the many narratives that accompanied the acute stage of the pandemic, not all received the same measure of attention. Though the problems resulting from inadequate resources and the inability to provide the necessary space and equipment to all Covid-19 sufferers were central to patients' wellbeing and cast doubt on whether Italy's healthcare system is as universalist as it still formally purports to be, they were given little visibility in the press. The nationally distributed newspapers began to address the question of rationing in March 2020, when SIAARTI, the Italian Society of Anesthesia, Analgesia, Resuscitation and Intensive Care, drafted a set of clinical ethics recommendations for allocating intensive care resources. Though the document was intended for the anesthesiologists working on the frontlines of the pandemic, the society also decided to make it public. The dilemmatic nature of the choices that clinics could be called upon to make thus became part of the public debate in very clear terms:

> Every physician may be forced to make split-second decisions which are ethically and clinically fraught: which patients will receive intensive care

treatment when the resources are not sufficient for the patients who are admitted.

(SIAARTI, 2020)

The recommendations suggest prioritizing "greatest life expectancy" over the other allocation principles that we mentioned earlier, such as the severity of the patients' condition or "first come, first served". Early reactions in the press evinced a certain shock, with an attempt to look beyond Italy's borders to confirm that what was happening in the country was also happening elsewhere. At the end of March, two editorials in *Avvenire*—the organ of the Episcopal Conference of Italy (CEI)—focused on the question of rationing resources, starting from a review of the very different choices made in a number of US states. The opinion pieces' major concern was with the risks that rationing can cause for the weaker segments of the population, such as the elderly and the disabled (Molinari, 2020a, 2020b). The *Corriere della Sera*—the country's largest-circulated newspaper—raised the issue of Italian rationing and its dilemmas, quoting an anesthesiologist who states that although the fact is not discussed publicly, rationing is an every-day practice in many overwhelmed intensive care units (Stella, 2020). A number of papers devoted at least one editorial to the issue, but the problem of scarce resources quickly disappeared from their pages, and its implications were never explored in any depth. Questions that have no straightforward, generally accept-able answers were skirted and even when raised were swiftly shunted into the background. The most extensive narratives of scarcity were those in the online debate, in particular on the websites dealing more directly with questions relating to health or citizen's and patient's rights. In the latter case, the narratives served largely as a vehicle for protest, often by counter-information groups predating the onset of the pandemic. By contrast, the mainstream dailies were much more uni-form in their choice (or neglect) of topics and in their difficulties in unpacking the implications. According to Affuso et al. (2020), the discourses conveyed by the media can be viewed from two main perspectives. The first distinguishes between different types of information media and specifically between the narratives that circulate in traditional media and those in the digital media and social networks (Tipaldo et al., 2020). The second observes discourses and how they change over time. Though they consider a limited time period, Affuso and colleagues find a clear change of pace a few weeks after the beginning of the emergency, when businesses reopened and people gradually returned to their normal movements at the beginning of June 2020. Earlier, in the first stage of the crisis during the first lockdown period from March 9 to May 18, the traditional media—as the main source of news—were "in unison in purveying a narrative centering on reassur-ance and shared commitment" (Affuso et al., 2020, p. 61), while the digital media and social networks celebrated new practices of sociality, from balcony concerts and posts taking an ironic slant on events, to ways of supporting remote social-izing as a means of overcoming feelings of isolation. Once the shock of the first weeks had passed, the second stage—confirming the need for a communication

approach rooted in the context, its transformations and the shifting interconnections between a variety of actors, motivations and content (Briggs & Hallin,
2016)—saw a distinct change in tone. Science was pictured as torn by opposing
views, while the institutions' responses were portrayed as confused and increasingly unable to arrive at a consensus about how and when to take action: media
coverage featured frequent conflicts between experts in an acerbic debate that did
nothing to inspire confidence in the often contradictory solutions that the institutions sought to put forward. The unity that marked the first stage gave way to a
cacophony of voices that testified to the rising uncertainty and impatience brought
by the pandemic, making the need to find answers all the more urgent.

8 Conclusions: who shall live?

In the foregoing pages, we reviewed some of the many complications that accompany healthcare decisions and in particular the difficulty of finding shared criteria
for setting priorities and meeting patients' legitimate demands. We also saw that
although there is a common tendency to believe that resource shortages are a problem that arises in emergencies, inequities in access, a lack of facilities and the
resulting rationing strategies are in reality endemic conditions that emergencies
can at most aggravate. The situation does not seem to have improved with the passing of time. In reflecting on the changes in the US healthcare system over the last
40 years, for example, Fuchs (2011) demonstrated on the basis of extensive empirical documentation that, for all the new technologies and undeniable advances that
have been made, the results achieved by medicine in recent decades have been
far from satisfactory, and that the problems of access, high cost of treatment and
poor health outcomes for large segments of the population remain substantially
the same as they have been for many years. This combination of epoch-making
advances and lingering structural problems seems typical of all Western countries:

> No country is as healthy as it could be; no country does as much for the sick
> as it is technically capable of doing. . . . The grim fact is that no nation is
> wealthy enough to avoid all avoidable deaths.
>
> (Fuchs, 2011, p. 17)

Sassen (2014a), in an equally wide-ranging reconstruction of the worldwide
dynamics of capitalism, uses the term *expulsions* to describe the massive increase
in the numbers of people who are left behind by processes of growth around
the world, victims of what she calls "predatory formations". Sassen puts espe-
cial emphasis on how expulsions have been particularly brutal in the processes
that have fueled the global economy in past decades, with little visibility and no
increase in the capacity to blunt these processes' negative impact. If these trends
are to be understood, Sassen maintains, we need analyses that can monitor the
new intensity of inequalities (Vicarelli & Spina, 2020), as well as a new language
and new conceptual categories for describing phenomena which are to a large

extent unfamiliar that can help shed light on their determinants. Demonstrating the need for a change of perspective, Sassen notes that processes of expulsion can also take place when phenomena that are apparently or partially positive intersect: "forms of knowledge and intelligence we respect and admire are often at the origin of long transaction chains that can end in simple expulsions" (2014a, p. 1). This, in a way, is what has happened in healthcare, where new diagnostic and treatment capabilities have in many countries been accompanied by an inadequate—and often increasingly so—ability to actually take care of patients and their needs, giving rise to new mechanisms of expulsion such as those associated with the high cost of new therapies or innovative diagnostic equipment.

The pandemic's spread in 2020, and its shattering effects, made the system's many contradictions and the knotty problems that still beset it all too tangible for patients (and more visible to the general public), exposing its fragility and showing how shaky the balance that sustained it had been and how seriously the risks generated by modernization processes were underestimated (Collier & Lakoff, 2014; Stiglitz, 2019; Lusardi & Tomelleri, 2020). The fact that in the spring and summer of 2020 the institutions had concentrated on the emergency aspects, without paying adequate attention to the system's long-standing structural shortcomings, to some extent made it less possible to recognize where responsibility lies for conditions that were years in the making. As we pointed out in Chapter 2, the state of the healthcare system is the result of decades of cuts, the growing privatization of care facilities and a determined and in some ways violent policy of scaling back welfare, healthcare and public assistance. These are choices whose origins date back at least to the 1980s in many Western countries, but whose consequences only began to be broadly apparent after a few decades, especially in emergencies such as the 2007 economic crash or the dramatic shortage of resources in the early stages of the 2020 pandemic. According to Pellizzoni (2020), much hinges on the capacity to anticipate the future, on being able to show that risks are under control, thus quieting the anxieties that well up when uncertainties cannot be dispelled by attempting to present the choices that are (or will be) necessary to make as inevitable. The concept of preparedness thus becomes central as does the ability to make the political choices entailed by preparedness seem to be techniques. As regards the ability to produce a certain concrete picture of the future and demonstrate that it is inevitable, politics' task thus calls for continual adjustment and adaptation:

> [P]reparedness points to developing capacities for governing a co-evolving dynamic of action and reaction, attack and counter-attack. It points to the modulation of a crisis that, more than leading to resolution, requires constant handling, subtle managerial abilities.
>
> (Pellizzoni, 2020, p. 47)

These managerial abilities, however, cannot escape the possibility that the outcomes may diverge. And as we have seen, we cannot promise to save all lives (nor can all such promises be kept), and some will have to face a more uncertain fate than others:

> This means that any type of anticipatory action will only provide relief, or promise to provide relief, to a valued life, not necessarily all of life. Certain lives may have to be abandoned, damaged or destroyed in order to protect, save or care for life.
>
> (Anderson, 2010, p. 780)

Allocative choices seem to be able to produce certain courses of action and to make decisions, and their horizon of possibilities appears inevitable. But as Sassen reminds us, "These expulsions don't simply happen; they are made" (2014b). They thus do not spring randomly from events beyond our control—where the most we can do is try to keep the consequences from getting out of hand—but are the political outcome of a certain conception of the world, a certain picture of the future, of past choices which may or may not have been made to prepare us for that future world (Fourcade, 2017).

Communication has a central role in these dynamics. The narratives that take shape (or that are intentionally constructed) are much more than simple reports showing, more or less accurately, what is going on: they are the means of normalizing courses of action, making the future horizons they paint acceptable to a degree. If the attention to value production[9] (Gallino, 2011) in such crucial areas as healthcare is to be preserved and its nature as a public good be developed—and here we come to our last point—transparency and public discussion are particularly important. And yet, these are precisely the conditions we have seen to be lacking in areas that "do not stand the light of day". Thus, despite the uncertainty of information and its inherently ambiguous nature, aspects we will turn to in the next chapter, developing informed communication resources and a well-supported public discourse seems more necessary than ever. It is undeniably difficult to find consensus solutions and provide patients and the community with precise information. But this must not be an alibi for abandoning the search for feasible solutions that seek a better balance of power between all players. As Sen reminds us, the game is by no means over, but we must be aware that:

> Not only is the force of public discussion one of the correlates of democracy, with an extensive reach, but its cultivation can also make democracy itself function better.
>
> (1999, p. 158)

Notes

1 In the 1990s, after extensive discussion among the experts followed by a ballot referendum, the state of Oregon decided to maintain its utilitarian approach to rationing decisions, extending cost–benefit analysis to prioritizing a larger set of procedures. For an

overview of the most recent developments, see https://sharedsystems.dhsoha.state.or.us/DHSForms/Served/le2288R.pdf

2 www.economist.com/leaders/2020/04/02/covid-19-presents-stark-choices-between-life-death-and-the-economy

3 Elster uses the term principle "to designate any general conception of how the scarce good is to be allocated" (1992, p. 62).

4 According to some scholars, the fact that the obviousness of stigmatization fails to be recognized and countered even by care providers also depends on the almost complete lack of medical education programs that, in addition to teaching clinical skills, devote space to moral concepts and the role of justice, with the result that there is little awareness of the their wide-ranging implications in clinical practice (Coulehan et al., 2003).

5 The purported link between mothering and autism is emblematic of the misattribution of the causes that can lead to the development of a disease. The mothers of autistic children have long been accused of having brought the condition about through their unaffectionate behavior. Though research has shown this hypothesis to be groundless, women who have been branded as "refrigerator mothers" continue to find themselves in the unenviable position of having to deal with complex symptoms while simultaneously being blamed for causing them (Jordynn, 2014).

6 According to the Disability Rights Education & Defense Fund: "Virtually all healthcare providers in the United States are subject to the disability nondiscrimination mandates of the ADA [American with Disabilities Act], Section 504, and/or Section 1557 of the ACA [Affordable Care Act]" (DREDF, 2020). These laws prohibit the denial of care on the basis of disability to an individual who would benefit from it.

7 Disaster medicine is a medical specialization that provides appropriate emergency responses following natural disasters or catastrophes of various kinds. In addition to identifying the organizational and practical tools needed to deal with emergencies, it also addresses disaster preparedness and preventive approaches to the dilemmas that must be faced.

8 An earlier version of the last two sections of the chapter was published in: N. Bosco (2021). "Who Shall Live? Discorsi pubblici e criteri di razionalizzazione ai tempi del Covid-19". In A. R. Favretto, A. Maturo, & S. Tomelleri (Eds.), *L'impatto sociale del Covid-19*. Milano: Franco Angeli, 263–272.

9 Gallino distinguishes between *value production*, where a certain area is valued and taken care of for the benefit of the community, and *value extraction*, which is the mark of the predatory approach taken by capitalism in the stage he calls finance capitalism: "a mega-machine developed in the last few decades in order to maximize and accumulate, in the form of both capital and power, the value that can be extracted from the maximum number of human beings and from ecosystems" (2011, p. 5).

References

Abbott, A. (2003). *Methods of Discovery. Heuristics for the Social Sciences*. New York: W.W. Norton & Company, Inc.

Affuso, O., Agodi, M. C., & Ceravolo, F. A. (2020). Scienza, expertise e senso comune: dimensioni simboliche e sociomateriali della pandemia, *AIS Journal of Sociology, 16*, 57–68. https://doi.org/10.1485/2281-2652-202016-4.

Anderson, B. (2010). Preemption, Precaution, Preparedness: Anticipatory Action and Future Geographies. *Progress in Human Geography, 34*(6), 777–798. https://doi.org/10.1177/0309132510362600.

Arlotti, M., & Ranci, C. (2020). *La strage nascosta. Cosa è accaduto nelle residenze per anziani durante la pandemia*. Laboratorio di Politiche Sociali. Politecnico di Milano. www.lps.polimi.it/?p=3592.

Batsch, N. L., Mittelman, M. S., & Alzheimer's Disease International. (2012). *Overcoming the Stigma of Dementia*. World Alzheimer Report 2012. www.alz.co.uk/research/WorldAlzheimerReport2012.pdf.

Beckford, M. (2008). Baroness Warnock: Dementia Sufferers May Have a 'Duty to Die'. *The Telegraph*, 18 September. www.telegraph.co.uk/news/uknews/2983652/Baroness-Warnock-Dementia-sufferers-may-have-a-duty-to-die.html.

Berney, L., Kelly, M., Doyal, L., Feder, G., Griffiths, C., & Jones, I. R. (2005). Ethical Principles and the Rationing of Health Care: A Qualitative Study in General Practice. *The British Journal of General Practice*, *55*(517), 620–625. https://bjgp.org/content/55/517/620.

Biddison, E. L. D., Faden, R., Gwon, H. S., Mareiniss, D. P., Regenberg, A. C., Schoch-Spana, M., Schwartz, J., & Toner, E. S. (2019). Too Many Patients . . . A Framework to Guide Statewide Allocation of Scarce Mechanical Ventilation During Disasters. *Chest*, *155*(4), 848–854. https://doi.org/10.1016/j.chest.2018.09.025.

Biddison, E. L. D., Gwon, H. S., Schoch-Spana, M., et al. (2018). Scarce Resource Allocation During Disasters: A Mixed-Method Community Engagement Study, *Chest*, *153*(1), 187–195. https://doi.org/10.1016/j.chest.2017.08.001.

Bobbio, L. (Ed.). (2013). *La qualità della deliberazione. Processi dialogici tra cittadini*. Roma: Carocci Editore.

Bobbio, L., Pomatto, G., & Seddone, A. (2015). Quando la politica soffoca le politiche. Una ricerca su media e politiche pubbliche. *Stato e mercato*, *35*(3), 509–536. https://doi.org/10.1425/81608.

Bohman, J. (1998). The Coming of Age of Deliberative Democracy. *The Journal of Political Philosophy*, *6*(4), 400–425. https://doi.org/10.1111/1467-9760.00061.

Briggs, C. L., & Hallin, D. C. (2016). *Making Health Public. How News Coverage Is Remaking Media, Medicine, and Contemporary Life*. London and New York: Routledge.

Brown, R. C. H. (2019). Irresponsibly Infertile? Obesity, Efficiency, and Exclusion from Treatment. *Health Care Analysis*, *27*(2), 61–76. https://doi.org/10.1007/s10728-019-00366-w.

Buchanan, A. (1989). *Health-Care Delivery and Resource Allocation*. In Veatch, R. M. (Ed.), *Medical Ethics*. Boston: Jones & Barlett.

Calabresi, G., & Bobbit, P. (1978). *Tragic Choices*. New York: Norton.

Care Quality Commission. (2011). *Dignity and Nutrition Inspection Programme: National Overview*. London: CQC.

Chisholm, N., Briggs, K., & Askham, J. (2009). *Not NICE: Can PCTs Engage Patients and the Public in Commissioning New Health Technologies?* Oxford: Picker Institute.

Clavien, C., & Hurst, S. (2019). The Undeserving Sick? An Evaluation of Patients' Responsibility for Their Health Condition. *Cambridge Quarterly of Healthcare Ethics*, *29*. https://doi.org/10.1017/S0963180119000975.

Cohen, S. (2001). *States of Denial. Knowing About Atrocities and Suffering*. Hoboken, NJ: John Wiley & Sons.

Collier, S. J., & Lakoff, A. (2014). Vital Systems Security: Reflexive Biopolitics and the Government of Emergency. *Theory, Culture & Society*, *32*(2), 19–51. https://doi.org/10.1177/0263276413510050.

Cookson, R., & Dolan, P. (2000). Principles of Justice in Health Care Rationing. *Journal of Medical Ethics*, *26*, 323–329. https://doi.org/10.1136/jme.26.5.323.

Coulehan, J., Williams, P., Van McCrary, S., & Belling, C. (2003). The Best Lack All Conviction: Biomedical Ethics, Professionalism, and Social Responsibility. *Cambridge Quarterly of Healthcare Ethics*, *12*(1), 21–38. https://doi.org/10.1017/S0963180103121044.

Daniels, N., & Sabin, J. (2002). *Setting Limits Fairly: Can We Learn to Share Medical Resources?* New York: Oxford University Press.

De Stefano, E. (2008). *Eugenetica*. Enciclopedia della Scienza e della Tecnica. www.treccani.it/enciclopedia/eugenica_%28Enciclopedia-della-Scienza-e-della-Tecnica%29/.

Disability Rights Education & Defense Fund (DREDF). (2020). *Preventing Discrimination in the Treatment of COVID-19 Patients: The Illegality of Medical Rationing on the Basis of Disability*, 25 March. https://dredf.org/the-illegality-of-medical-rationing-on-the-basis-of-disability/.

Edmonds, D. (2014). *Would You Kill the Fat Man? The Trolley Problem and What Your Answer Tells Us About Right and Wrong*. Princeton: Princeton University Press.

Elster, J. (1992). *Local Justice. How Institutions Allocate Scarce Goods and Necessary Burdens*. New York: Russell Sage Foundation.

Emanuel, E. J., Persad, G., Upshur, R., Thome, B., Parker, M., Glickman, A., Zhang, C., Boyle, C., Smith, M., & Phillips, J. P. (2020). Fair Allocation of Scarce Medical Resources in the Time of Covid-19. *New England Journal of Medicine, 382*, 2049–2055. https://doi.org/10.1056/NEJMsb2005114.

Engel, G. L. (1977). The Need for a New Medical Model: A Challenge for Biomedicine. *Science, 196*(4286), 129–136. https://doi.org/10.1126/science.847460.

Feltri, S. (2020). Qual è il prezzo delle nostre vite. *Il Fatto Quotidiano*, 15 April.

Fourcade, M. (2017). The Fly and the Cookie: Alignment and Unhingement in 21st-Century Capitalism. *Socio-Economic Review, 15*(3), 661–678. https://doi.org/10.1093/ser/mwx032.

Fuchs, V. (2011). *Who Shall Live? Health, Economics and Social Choice*. Hackensack, NJ: World Scientific Publishing.

Gallino, L. (2011). *Finazcapitalismo. La civiltà del denaro in crisi*. Torino: Einaudi.

Ham, C., & Pickard, S. (1998). *Tragic Choices in Health Care*. London: The King's Fund.

Jones, I. R., Berney, L., Kelly, M., Doyal, L., Griffiths, C., Feder, G., Hillier, S., Rowlands, G., & Curtis, S. (2004). Is Patient Involvement Possible When Decisions Involve Scarce Resources? A Qualitative Study of Decision-Making in Primary Care. *Social Science & Medicine, 59*(1), 93–102. http://dx.doi.org/10.1016/j.socscimed.2003.10.007.

Jordynn, J. (2014). *Autism and Gender: From Refrigerator Mothers to Computer Geeks*. Urbana, Chicago and Springfield: University of Illinois Press.

Kahneman, D., & Tversky, A. (1984). Choices, Values and Frames. *American Psychologist, 39*(4), 341–350. https://pdfs.semanticscholar.org/44ea/b3013cb6c63a534570994c-9cffe3935ec7ed.pdf.

Kahn-Harris, K. (2018). *Denial: The Unspeakable Truth*. London: Notting Hill Editions.

Kevern, P. (2017). Why Are We So Afraid of Dementia? *The Conversation*, 12 September. https://theconversation.com/why-are-we-so-afraid-of-dementia-83175.

Klein, R., & Maybin, J. (2012). *Thinking About Rationing*. London: The King's Fund. www.kingsfund.org.uk/sites/default/files/field/field_publication_file/Thinking-about-rationing-the-kings-fund-may-2012.pdf.

Knaak, S., Mantler, E., & Szeto, A. (2017). Mental Illness-Related Stigma in Healthcare: Barriers to Access and Care and Evidence-Based Solutions. *Healthcare Management Forum, 30*(2), 111–116. https://doi.org/10.1177/0840470416679413.

Koonin, L. M., Pillai, S., Kahn, E. B., Moulia, D., & Patel, A. (2020). Strategies to Inform Allocation of Stockpiled Ventilators to Healthcare Facilities During a Pandemic. *Health Security, 18*(2), 69–74. https://doi.org/10.1089/hs.2020.0028.

Lupton, D. (1993). Risk as Moral Danger: The Social and Political Functions of Risk Discourse in Public Health. *International Journal of Health Services*, *23*(3), 425–435. https://doi.org/10.2190%2F16AY-E2GC-DFLD-51X2.

Lusardi, R., & Tomelleri, S. (2020). Algoritmi, cigni neri e virus: la crisi della pianificazione sociale nella modernità avanzata. *AIS Journal of Sociology*, *16*, 23–38. https://doi.org/10.1485/2281-2652-202016-2.

Marroni, C. A., Fleck, A. M., Jr, Fernandes, S. A., Galant, L. H., Mucenic, M., de Mattos Meine, M. H., Mariante-Neto, G., & Brandão, A. (2018). Liver Transplantation and Alcoholic Liver Disease: History, Controversies, and Considerations. *World Journal of Gastroenterology*, *24*(26), 2785–2805. https://doi.org/10.3748/wjg.v24.i26.2785.

Molinari, E. (2020a). Virus. Usa, "niente respiratori per i disablili". Più di 10 Stati scelgono chi salvare. *Avvenire.it*, 25 March. www.avvenire.it/mondo/pagine/niente-respiratori-per-i-disabili-pi-di-10-stati-scelgono-chi-salvare.

Molinari, E. (2020b). Polemica. Disabili non meritevoli di respiratori. Gli Usa si ribellano: valoreprezioso. *Avvenire.it*, 27 March. www.avvenire.it/mondo/pagine/disabili-usa-senza-respiratore.

Niemeyer, S., & Dryzek, J. S. (2007). The Ends of Deliberation: Meta-Consensus and Inter-Subjective Rationality as Ideal Outcomes. *Swiss Political Science Review*, *13*(4), 497–526. https://researchprofiles.canberra.edu.au/en/publications/the-ends-of-deliberation-meta-consensus-and-inter-subjective-rati.

Pellizzoni, L. (2007). *Cosa significa deliberare? Promesse e problemi della democrazia deliberativa*. In Id. (Ed.), *La deliberazione pubblica*. Roma: Meltemi, 7–48.

Pellizzoni, L. (2020). The Time of Emergency. On the Governmental Logic of Preparedness. *AIS Journal of Sociology*, *16*, 39–54. https://doi.org/10.1485/2281-2652-202016-3.

Rawls, J. (1971). *A Theory of Justice*. Cambridge: Harvard University Press.

Regonini, G. (2005). Paradossi della democrazia deliberativa. *Stato e Mercato*, *73*, 3–31. www.jstor.org/stable/24650827.

Sabik, L. M., & Lie, R. K. (2008). Priority Setting in Health Care: Lessons from the Experiences of Eight Countries. *International Journal for Equity in Health*, *7*, 4. https://doi.org/10.1186/1475-9276-7-4.

Sassen, S. (2014a). *Expulsions: Brutality and Complexity in the Global Economy*. Cambridge, MA: Belknap Press—Harvard University Press.

Sassen, S. (2014b). The Language of Expulsion. *Truthout*. https://truthout.org/articles/the-language-of-expulsion/.

Sen, A. K. (1999). *Development as Freedom*. New York: Alfred A. Knopf, Inc.

SIAARTI. (2020). *Clinical Ethics Recommendations for the Allocation of Intensive Care Treatments in Exceptional, Resource-Limited Circumstances—Version 1*, 16 March. www.siaarti.it/SiteAssets/News/COVID19%20-%20documenti%20SIAARTI/SIAARTI%20-%20Covid-19%20-%20Clinical%20Ethics%20Reccomendations.pdf.

Stella, G. A. (2020). Coronavirus, la lotta per la vita e il diritto alla cura per anziani e disabili: "Non discriminateli". *Corriere.it*, 20 March. www.corriere.it/esteri/20_marzo_31/coronavirus-lotta-la-vita-diritto-cura-anziani-disabili-non-discriminateli-1aa9c874-738b-11ea-bc49-338bb9c7b205.shtml.

Stiglitz, J. (2019). *People, Power, and Profits: Progressive Capitalism for an Age of Discontent*. New York: Norton Company.

Tipaldo, G., Carriero, R., Bruno, F., Pasquettaz, G., & Rocutto, S. (2020). Parlare della pandemia su Facebook: un'analisi comparata del contenuto su dati generati dagli utenti a Bergamo, Milano e Padova. *Sociologia Italiana—AIS Journal of Sociology*, *16*, 141–164. https://doi.org/10.1485/2281-2652-202016-9.

Vicarelli, G., & Spina, E. (2020). Disuguaglianze e Servizio Sanitario Nazionale: una contraddizione irrisolvibile? *Politiche Sociali—Social Policies*, *1*, 77–102. https://doi.org/10.7389/97336.

Vineis, P., & Capri, S. (1994). *La salute non è una merce. Efficacia della medicina e politiche sanitarie*. Torino: Bollati Boringhieri.

Waeckerle, J. F., Lillibridge, S. R., Burkle, F. M., & Noji, E. K. (1994). Disaster Medicine: Challenges for Today. *Annals of Emergency Medicine*, *23*(4), 715–718. https://doi.org/10.1016/S0196-0644(94)70304-3.

Chapter 4

Images of health

Public discourse, information, ignorance and communication

As we saw in the conclusions to Chapter 3, the thorny questions in healthcare—the tragic choices that do not stand the light of day—are hard to bring out into the open, and just as hard to communicate. And yet, it is undeniably important to present a clear view of all the alternatives whenever decisions must be made that can have repercussions on the life of the community. Knowing what options are available and their underlying assumptions, crafting effective messages about them and ensuring that these messages are heard can help in basing decisions on due diligence and making their outcomes more readily acceptable. These are aspects that are all the more important when the objectives in question concern public health and strategies for improving it. Now, in our final chapter, a few more steps are needed to illustrate how the nexus between communication and health is formed and imagine routes that can lead to a better understanding of these links and reduce the distance between the public and the institutions.

In the following pages, we will attempt to bring a measure of order to what we have seen so far. The importance of explicit or implicit representations concerning health and the clarity—or confusion—that they can bring urge greater attention to the nature of the ideas thus circulated and the mechanisms that can help us understand what remains, undiscussed, in the shadows. Starting from the different—and often overlapping—ideas of what science is and what we can expect from it that have come and gone over the years, we will focus our attention on what can be observed today and, above all, on what does not become visible and on some of the reasons that certain issues we might hope to see represented—were we to take a purely rational view of the relationship between health and communication—are never addressed.

1 Discourses on a continuum between efficacy and exclusion

The conceptions and representations of health and illness have a lengthy history, a history enmeshed and intertwined with our ideas about science, its transformations, the ups and downs in its credibility over the ages and the credibility of the actors on the scientific stage. Never, before the pandemic that swept the world

DOI: 10.4324/9780367854515-5

in 2020, had we been exposed to so many representations of healthcare systems and their functions, the goals they pursue and the targets they hit, their failures, their shortcomings and how they could be overcome. As in many other important areas—that of the economic choices needed to tackle the crisis, for example—the pandemic affected what was considered sayable, making certain aspects of the situation natural (or naturalizing them) and censuring others. Many topics did not receive the attention that their centrality—not least for the millions of patients around the globe who are bearing the consequences—would have required. As the following pages will show, the reasons these issues were ignored or neglected stem from particular combinations of heterogeneous factors. For example, as we saw in Chapter 3, the problems resulting from healthcare rationing strategies did not enter the public debate, as they were mentioned almost in passing and quickly shoved aside. Likewise, the pandemic's toll on patients with non-Covid-related disease or who were still waiting for a diagnosis was not given sufficient visibility, even though delays and postponements in doctor's appointments, testing and surgical procedures (Rosenbaum, 2020) and the suspension of many screening programs (Armaroli et al., 2020) have had difficult, and at times dramatic, consequences for thousands of people. Moreover, though there is a rich and growing literature on the increase in health inequalities between patients within and across countries (in vaccine availability, for instance) and the risks this can bring, few of its findings have found their way into the public discourse and the policy agenda (Bambra et al., 2020; Teixeira da Silva, 2020; Jensen et al., 2021).

Intentionally or otherwise, these narratives—and the silences, the silences that speak volumes which are part of the narratives (Bosco, 2012; Scott, 2018)—have spawned different conceptions of medicine and the relationships between institutions and the public which have in turn influenced the options for patient care. Even in times less fraught than these, what the institutions see fit to communicate about healthcare and the chances that the information they circulate will lead to an outcome of some kind raises complex questions.

Before coming to the nub of what we can learn from how the healthcare issues that will receive attention are selected, it should be pointed out that there is no such thing as entirely unambiguous communication. It is never easy to gauge whether any communication process has reached the goals it set out to achieve or, conversely, has led to other unforeseen or unwanted outcomes. Nor is it a simple matter to collect evidence in order to understand whether the outcomes, intentional or otherwise, have resulted from what has been done, or from other concomitant circumstances that have nothing to do with the communication methods that were used (Martini & Falletti, 2005). For example, if a communication campaign about the dangers of nuclear power plants had been carried out immediately before the Chernobyl meltdown in 1986, it would have been extremely difficult to determine if and to what extent any increase in the public's perception of the risks was correlated with the campaign. In any case, we have long known that the effects of information campaigns about complex issues are often rather limited, even if the issues they address involve problems that can be considered significant from many standpoints (Hyman & Sheatsley, 1947). Methodological problems aside, the efficacy of communication strategies is frequently overestimated, just as it is by no means automatic that experts and institutions will have coordinated information at their disposal, and will be able to convey it fittingly. Institutions not infrequently fall victim to the "curse of knowledge" (Newton, 1990, in Heath, 2003), where their own knowledge of a subject makes them forget that not everyone is similarly well-informed. This leads them to be overconfident about their audience's ability to understand and retain the content of their messaging, taking for granted that others will make the effort to decode it. The experiment that illustrated the workings of this mechanism consisted of asking one group of people to tap out the rhythm of well-known songs with their fingers, and another group of people to guess what song it was. Before the experiment started, the "tappers" were asked to predict how often the "listeners" would guess correctly. The tappers' predictions turned out to be wildly inaccurate: while they had expected that the songs would be identified 50% of the time, the listeners guessed only 2.5% of the songs correctly, or three times out of 120. When we have been "cursed" by knowledge, or in other words, we intend to convey something that seems obvious and understandable to us, like how a song we are tapping out sounds in our own heads, it becomes extremely difficult to put ourselves in the shoes of someone who is not privy to this knowledge—and consequently hears only an unmusical series of taps. Clearly, if institutions believe they have communicated clearly and carefully but the public does not get the message, they could blame the public for what was in fact an effect of the curse of knowledge, with all of the worrisome repercussions that this can have on mutual trust or the ability to understand what went wrong.

For example, institutions may overestimate the likelihood that people will translate the information they have been given into actual conduct. A study of 20 years of public health efforts in the United Kingdom to promote responsible antibiotic use and mitigate antimicrobial resistance (AMR)—or in other words the growing inefficacy of currently available antibiotics—led to findings that were to some extent unexpected. For instance, there continues to be widespread ignorance about when antibiotics should be used even among people who had been exposed to public health messaging.

And confirming what has long been known (Rosenstock, 1974), it was also found that even those who had gained more specific knowledge about antibiotics' action neither changed their behavior as hoped nor reduced their use of antibiotics (Will, 2020). Indeed, having positive attitudes about a given topic (the damage wrought by heavy drinking, for example) does not necessarily mean that this information will be translated into behavior which is in fact consistent with it (drinking less, or not drinking at all). As a result, identifying the frequently undesired (or at least suboptimal) effects of the communication process is far from straightforward (Stacy et al., 1994; Clapp et al., 2003; van Doorn et al., 2007). In addition to the assumptions of the social and cultural environment in which communication circulates, any consideration of its efficacy hinges, first, on the credibility granted to science and its practitioners and on the perceptions of scientists themselves (Scamuzzi & Tipaldo, 2015). To get our bearings here, it is thus useful to dig deeper into the nature of discourses about health, of the conceptions regarded as legitimate and how they vary, because the fact that their meanings become naturalized tends to blind us to just how partial our purview is. As a result, we are often unable to understand the underlying mechanisms, so we cannot even imagine what the alternatives for improvement might be. This is a point that bears repeating because, as we have often had occasion to emphasize, it involves an awareness that is almost impossible to retain and must thus be returned to again and again.

Though the complications we have described do not depend on the actors' intentions, we must also remember that—as Foucault points out—the *ordre du discours*, or the concrete shape that discourse takes, is often the outcome of specific kinds of subjection, with a broad streak of exclusion inevitably running through them:

> [N]ot all the regions of discourse are equally open and penetrable; some of them are largely forbidden (they are differentiated and differentiating), while others seem to be almost open to all winds and put at the disposal of every speaking subject, without prior restrictions.
> (Foucault, 1971, English translation 1981, p. 62)

Depending on the circumstances, these procedures of exclusion can shape practices that have more to do with the exercise of power than with the content of a dispute. Likewise, not all discourses may enjoy the same legitimacy, or their legitimacy may not hold firm over time: certain issues simply remain outside any dialectical exchange and cannot be named or faced on the public stage (the *taboo on the object of* speech), as appears to be the case of the decisions about who will be saved, which we discussed in Chapter 3. Foucault notes that there is also a second procedure or system of exclusion; the fact that not everyone has the same power of speech, *the privileged or exclusive right of the speaking subject.* This is nothing new; history is liberally sprinkled with clashes between opposing conceptions of the world—rules and/or customs—that grant certain parties the right to name reality to their liking and impose their own interpretations (Hirshman, 1991). Certain ideas and practices, taken for granted in the past, at a certain point become less obvious, whether through the passage of time, new knowledge, new ideas of what is most appropriate or *normal* (Canguilhem, 1966) or because the conceptions of power and who holds it have changed. That the spotlight is on the role of the speaker and not the content of the speech alters the outcomes of the discourse and shifts the resulting equilibria (Bourdieu, 1982). The performative power of utterances—words' capacity to function and act concretely—exists even when the logical connection between words and the outcomes of discourse is not immediately apparent (Austin, 1962; Butler, 1997). These dynamics are not exclusive to the sphere of science, which we will discuss in greater detail later in this chapter. Rather, they reflect the more general need to normalize and combat the uncertainty that comes with the territory for human beings and the societies they form. Foucault offers the following description of the—to us, at least, rather bizarre—definition of what judicial truth meant at the end of the eighteenth century and the implicit assumptions about defendants' guilt:

> [C]lassical law said: if the sum does not add up to that minimum degree of proof on the basis of which the full and entire penalty can be applied, if the addition remains in some way uncertain, if there is simply three-quarters proof and not a full proof in the total sum, nevertheless this does not mean that one should not punish. To a three-quarters proof corresponds a three-quarters penalty, to a semi-proof, a semi-penalty. In other words, one is not suspected with impunity. The least element of proof, or, in any case, a certain element of proof, will be enough to entail a certain element of penalty.
>
> (Foucault, 1999, English translation 2003, p. 7)

Proofs were assembled and weighted in a hierarchy of "complete proofs and incomplete proofs, full proofs and semifull proofs, whole proofs and half proofs, indications and cavils". It was not necessary to provide an empirically grounded demonstration of the guilt of someone accused of a given crime, but to apply rules and procedures established by tradition and regarded as indisputable. The fact that it was not possible to follow objective procedures in order to apply the law impartially and determine whether the defendant was indeed guilty seems not to have prevented this "arithmetic of proof" from becoming binding and freighted with consequences, nor does it appear to have been seen as a problem (except for the poor unfortunates in the dock). Foucault's example suggests that in order to decode the relationship between representations, the visibility of issues and the chances they will gain ground, we must go beyond a narrow focus on the divide between the experts' rationality and the public's lack of knowledge. And this is what we propose to do in the following pages.

2 Public health and the representations and conceptions of health

The assumptions about the foundations of scientific knowledge vary widely. But the point that interests us here has little to do with the epistemological discussions of science's objectivity.

Once again, two seemingly secondary factors draw our attention; the first is that certain assumptions continue to enjoy credibility even though the empirical evidence is against them (Heath, 2003; Heath & Heath, 2007); the second has to do with the difficulty in recognizing the often contingent character of what we hold to be true (D'Agostini, 2010; Ferraris, 2017). Not even science—commonly considered the very emblem of rationality—seems exempt from the tendency to label constructs as true without verifying their basis in fact and the resulting difficulty of determining what ought to presented in the broader social context. It must, however, be borne in mind that—given the normative force of institutions or the weight of majority views in a community of individuals—images, ideas and representations can gain sway and influence the choice of the goals to be pursued and many other aspects. In healthcare, these aspects can include patients' perceptions of their condition, patient/caregiver relations or the recognition given to health professionals, all of which thus call for close attention. As we look at the representations of health, it is not enough to determine how reliable the information being circulated may be; we must also observe the underlying mechanisms, e.g., the relationship between those who hold the power of speech and the heterogeneous publics to whom discourses are addressed or these representations' effects on the mutual expectations of audience and actors in the healthcare theater. As Farre & Rapley emphasize, "The importance of how the object of medical work is conceptualised (i.e., in terms of disease or illness) lies in the fact that such definition is paramount to understand the boundaries and scope of responsibility associated with such work" (2017, p. 2). Given that the conceptions of health and illness are not cultural invariants, interest also attaches to the often murky process of choosing the issues which are considered to deserve attention, and why certain topics pop up everywhere while others linger in the background.

How we define health, the language we use to talk about it and the information that circulates open onto different panoramas of possibility and different roads for bringing our choices to life. At the macro level, these roads are the politics and the policies that, respectively, decide on the goals and determine what steps are necessary to achieve them. At the micro level, exploring these alternative panoramas can help us redefine our relationship with the world. When disease strikes, for example, ill people have to learn "to think differently", because they can no longer rely on the destination and map they had used to navigate and must reinvent their daily lives and reframe their expectations (Frank, 2013). But "re-orienting the vision of healthcare providers away from a biomedical and reductionist view of patienthood, towards a more holistic understanding of the meanings of illness for those who experience it" (Seale, 2003, p. 513) is not free from complications. Heterogeneity itself can be a source of confusion, as it is often accompanied by the spread of contradictory or even intentionally misleading information (Wang et al., 2019) which may be difficult to winnow out.

However important they may be, the representations that circulate in society in the form of "culturally available narratives, stories, scripts, discourses, systems of knowledge or, in a more politically oriented analyses, ideologies" (Seale, 2003, p. 514) do not always help us determine what content and information are reasonably reliable. There are so many of them that they can at best enable us to posit provisional and contingent truths that reflect the viewpoints, interests and varyingly partial knowledge of those who decide what content will be presented. On the other hand, this heterogeneity is beneficial inasmuch as it serves up an enormous menu of options and resources, in the form of ideas, repertoires of action and "cultural scripts" that can include "depictions of what it is like to be sick, what causes illness, health and cure, how healthcare providers behave (or ought to) and the nature of health policies and their impact" (Seale, 2003, p. 514). In addition, this array of representations can shine a light on the society we live in, on what we value, on how we deal with uncertainty and come to grips with what we have decided are the problem, and what we propose to do about them (Blumer, 1971; Golding & Middleton, 1982; Gusfield, 1989; Lupton, 1993).

2.1 Defining health

Words, as we have pointed out several times, are not neutral. And the attempts to reconstruct what we think ought to fall under the heading of health testify to the variability and ambiguities that speech involves, and to the responsibility of the speaker, especially if the speaker represents an institution (Bianchi, 2021). Even the definition presented in the Constitution of the World Health Organization, however much we may agree with its spirit, is not entirely free from contradictions. Health here is defined as "a state of complete physical, mental and social well-being and not merely the absence of infirmity"[1] which, by not considering only the physiological aspects—as is commonly done from an organicist perspective—broke new ground because "it made explicit that disease and infirmity, when isolated from subjective experience, are inadequate to qualify health" (Saracci, 1997, p. 1409). Nevertheless, throwing open the door to unidentified social and psychological aspects raises a number of unanswered questions. It has been pointed out, for instance, that equating health with a state of complete well-being is unrealistic and that no one would qualify as healthy under this definition: a still-symptomless or undiagnosed disease could be mistakenly interpreted as health, with all the consequences this could entail. All prevention strategies, like the screening campaigns that many countries invite segments of the population to participate in, are based on the assumption that there is a real distinction between health and well-being that does not depend solely on individuals' perceptions of their state.

Two further aspects of the WHO definition have drawn criticism: first, its vagueness makes it difficult to find the best ways to promote the population's health or monitor trends (Ciofi, 2015). Second, thinking of health as a complete state and ignoring the fact that the relationship between health and illness is not necessarily binary, but a process, does not help us identify and circumscribe the problems that must be tackled or formulate policies for dealing with them (Huber et al., 2011). In connection with this latter aspect, the inadequacy of a dichotomous contrast between health and illness has been thrown into even sharper relief in the period since the WHO definition was introduced by the exponential rise in the numbers of people living with chronic disease, who can oscillate between the two poles for long periods in forms that are hard to predict (Badash et al., 2017).

Lastly, it should be noted that the WHO definition's embrace of a range of aspects that went beyond the merely physiological was not the straightforward and consensus-driven result of a steady increase in knowledge concerning the multifactorial nature of health. In the same years that the WHO proposed its definition,

Parsons' (1951) structural-functionalist model was fast gaining headway in the United States: though it did not deny the relational dimension of illness, Parsons' model considered it as deviance which prevents people from carrying out some or all of their normal social duties, accentuating illness' dysfunctional aspects and the need to restore equilibrium. Other theoretical and analytical perspectives were also part of the same historical moment: the views associated with medical anthropology, which see the healthcare system as the result of cross-fertilization between popular conceptions and professional knowledge, or the phenomenological approaches which attach increasing importance to patients' lived experience, to the subjective meaning they assign to illness and to the caregiving tasks performed outside the healthcare system (Kleinman et al., 1978; Lidler, 1979). A few short years later, symbolic interactionism and ethnomethodology pointed to the variable and socially constructed aspects of being ill and noted that patients follow specific *moral careers* going well beyond the biological aspects (Goffman, 1961). From this perspective, illness is scrutinized in terms of changes that take place over time as conditions vary and on the basis of the relational dynamics in the everyday interactions between everyone involved in all of illness' stages, death included (Glaser & Strauss, 1965). Such aspects as the social meaning of illness, patients' experiences and medical knowledge itself—all heavily dependent on contexts and relationships—differ from time to time in how they are recognized and legitimized (Freidson, 1970). How the symptoms of a certain illness present and are diagnosed and labeled, for example, depend both on the patients' experience and on the treatment options (Conrad & Barker, 2010).

What concerns us most here are not the details of each perspective, but the wide range and frequent overlapping of approaches whose only constant seems to be how they vary, in ways that far predate modern ideas of health. As Badash and colleagues remind us, holistic and societal ideas of health were already current in the very remote past—since the fifth century BCE—in Hippocrates' drive to separate "Greek medicine from magical and religious beliefs and establish the relationship between environmental/personal cleanliness and the origin of disease", and in the first century BCE, when Galen's thinking contributed to the spread of a more holistic idea of health that considered the patient's entire condition, "including mental and emotional states" (2017, p. 3).

The changes that have taken place over time thus cannot be described as the product of increasing medical knowledge, under the (mistaken) impression that such an increase could not fail to bring about a convergence in how sickness and health are viewed. Even in our own day, many heterogeneous ideas persist, although certain approaches have become naturalized to the point that they seem to predominate, masking what is in fact a plurality of perspectives. For example, Foucault (1963, English translation, 1973) notes that medicine began to take a logical rational perspective toward the end of the eighteenth century. In the following centuries, this approach was given new impetus by the growth of clinical and diagnostic skills, the innovations in surgery brought about by new techniques for disinfection and sterilization, the development of anesthesiology, the birth of epidemiology and new statistical and sampling methods that provided insights into the spread of diseases and treatment outcomes (Neresini, 2001). This was when the biomedical model came into its own: "It assumes disease to be fully accounted for by deviations from the norm of measurable biological (somatic) variables" (Engel, 1977, p. 196). Illness is thus a break from the organism's earlier equilibrium, which treatment is intended to reinstate. The social sciences, or at least some of their exponents, took up this perspective and contributed to reinforcing it. Parsons' functionalist model, for example, holds that the social system is in a continual tension toward equilibrium and, as Frank notes, even the idea of illness as something that throws the organism off-kilter presupposes that equilibrium must be restored: "Parson's modernist 'sick role' carries the expectation that ill people get well, cease to be patients, and return to their normal obligations" (Frank, 2013, p. 9). Healthcare itself was transformed to serve this function of restoring sick bodies to equilibrium, through the increasing specialization of roles, the birth of hospitals, the development of a specific organization of work and the testing of treatments and diagnostic procedures. If health is considered to depend essentially on organic conditions, it follows that attention should focus on the physiology of each individual organ in order to restore its function. The professionalization of the medical class through specialized educational programs is a response to this need for increasingly specific and sectorialized skills. And this, as Neresini (2001) points out, is encouraged by—and at the same time fuels—the growing specialization of knowledge and the increasing distance from a set of traditional healing practices now considered anything but scientific. Though it has been criticized for its biological reductionism, the biomedical model undoubtedly owes its success to its many real or attributed achievements[2] (Colombo & Rebughini, 2003).

In the late 1980s, evidence-based medicine began to build on the growing ability to establish empirically grounded causal links, and has gone from strength to strength down to our own. While the philosophical and epistemological origins of this approach date to the late 1800s, it is thanks to its increasing institutionalization—starting with the work of Cochrane (1972) and other scholars at the end of the 1960s, followed by the intensified efforts in medical education and organization in the 1990s (Sackett et al., 1996)—that it has been able to present itself as the model that best embodies objective knowledge and, consequently, real science (Smith & Rennie, 2014). While the ideas about science and possible treatment methods have historically been quite variable, divergent concepts and practices are no longer considered to be an asset or a source of stimulus. Rather, they are seen as potentially risky, apt to fuel confusion and—accordingly—to be quashed to make way for the mounting dominance of real science, sworn enemy of any form of treatment rooted in superstition or magical thinking. Thus, in the early twentieth century, "the scientific outlook, logical and rational, consolidated its position to become the prime means of knowing and producing truth" (Colombo & Rebughini, 2003, p. 17).

Alongside the more codified and respectable forms of knowledge, however, there has never been a lack of heterogeneous approaches to health whose failure to gain legitimacy has often been accompanied by a general whittling away of the ability to determine what forms of treatment can best meet the needs of a variegated population of patients. Osteopathy, founded in 1874 by Andrew Taylor Still, is a curious amalgam of certain assumptions taken from the conventional idea of treatment and principles that depart from it dramatically (Colombo & Rebughini, 2003). We thus find the notion—shared with the biomedical model—that alterations in the organism can be rectified by the healer—the osteopath in this case—but unlike the biomedical model, osteopathy holds that restoring equilibrium does not hinge on the illness per se and its symptoms but on the patient's overall condition, which the healer must thus bear well in mind. Interestingly, the refusal to regard clinical approaches that depart from the methods of conventional medicine as scientific has in this case also led to the rejection of a broader view of illness and treatment.

3 The analytical space: a proposal

Constitutively, science deals in provisional truths whose nature changes as new knowledge is gained. Many ideas that seem good then show themselves—as conditions change and time passes—to be naïve, unfounded or just plain wrong (Heath & Heath, 2007). Dominant narratives often seem to assume a linear idea of progress, inevitably bringing a greater capacity to investigate reality and identify the causal mechanism behind problems, and thus master them. The changes brought by tools for observing reality that were not available in the past or new skills in gathering information, however, tell only part of the story. A different narrative describes far less linear processes, where the contrast between official science and alternative paradigms is not so clear-cut that only ideas proven to be robustly well-founded can prevail. In this second set of circumstances, understanding why certain perspectives based on strong evidence are not accepted while others resting on far shakier ground continue to be considered credible requires us to look at aspects that cannot be readily grasped in terms of the march of progress. We must thus search for signs, not only of advances and new knowledge but also of the new waves and ripples in the cultural conceptions of science and its achievements in the settings where they arise and in the power relationships they entail. Digging down into current ideas about science—and their uneven acceptance—requires us to draw on the social as well as the physical sciences. But it should be emphasized that our aims here are circumscribed. We will limit ourselves to observing how the different perspectives cover a territory that is too broad to give us any single view of what science is or what it should do, without lapsing into attitudes that deny its validity and methods. Once again, we must stress that these perspectives have not followed each other in an orderly, linear sequence and that myriad and often contradictory approaches and conceptions have continued to vie with each other. The idea is that a close look at the coexistence of, and the confusion between, the different narratives of health and the repercussions on their public aspects can spark curiosity about present-day dynamics and draw attention to the many areas that still require clarification.

Understanding the mechanisms that determine how health is defined and who holds the responsibilities associated with it thus calls for a more panoramic vision. To go beyond interpretations that limit themselves to setting science against pseudoscience—and to investigate their implications for communication—we propose that the analytical space should be expanded. As this is simply a proposal, our intention is to encourage further reflection about the dimensions involved in analyzing discourses on science and healthcare. Such categorical contrasts as true/false, right/wrong, better/worse are poor tools for understanding the whys and wherefores of the field we are dealing with here and, presumably, of many others. This is not just because they entail judgments whose origins are sometimes difficult to find (as we saw for health service rankings in Chapter 1) but also because the fact that they implicitly assign responsibility can lead to blaming precisely those people—the patients—who bear the burden of illness and are least able to cope with it, as we found in Chapter 3.

As should be clear from the foregoing pages, healthcare and its outcomes depend on a broad set of combined conditions that cannot be understood if we think only in terms of two binary opposites: rationality, said to be the domain of science and experts; and irrationality, or lack of information on the part of the public. Taking a broader view means that we must sharpen our focus on the heterogeneity of the actors involved, and their differing outlooks and values, in order to increase community engagement in public health matters (Simis et al., 2016).

In our attempt to expand the analytical space, we have thus drawn up a matrix with two intersecting dimensions (Table 4.1). The first dimension runs from science to anti-scientism, the second from binding normative conceptions emanating from authority at one pole to plural conceptions at the other. We will start from the first. Science can be considered the set of theoretical and empirical conceptions that share rules and principles for observing reality and presuppose a specific definition of methods whereby reality can be analyzed. Broad though the scientific domain is, it does, however, have certain basic coordinates in common, and, as Beyerstein emphasizes, science "is not a grab-bag of immutable facts, but rather a way of asking questions and evaluating possible answers" (1996, p. 2).

As we will see, anti-scientism also channels very different perspectives, held together by their refusal to believe that the fundamental principles of science are universal and absolute. It thus includes conceptions that deny science's validity and oppose its pursuit, citing the risks that could ensue, as well as others that do not reject the existence of science as such, but argue that its role is less central than that of other less measurable and codifiable aspects of reality (Peters, 2020), or object to how science has been institutionalized, muzzling other voices. What these stances and their further expressions have in common is their rejection of methods that claim to have been codified, validated and established once and for all, holding that this is either impossible or risky.

The two poles of the second dimension are equally multifaceted: binding normative conceptions can—as we will see—originate with actors inside or outside the realm of science, in very different ways, times and places. In all cases, though, there is an authority of some kind who is able to dictate what the conception will be by relying on persuasive or manipulative strategies (Van Dijk, 2006) or other coercive methods that range from moral sanctions to violence at their most extreme. Moreover, it is assumed that there is only one authority who can say what *truth* is, just as there is only one truth that must be defended by every means from false interpretations, whatever the intentions that brought these interpretations to the fore. For its part, the pole of plural conceptions consists, by definition, of a plurality. What ties these conceptions together is that none seeks to set limits on definitions and constructs: all encourage the circulation and exploration of ideas, leaving freedom of choice as to what will be done. Efforts to limit the courses of action can be viewed with suspicion, as stemming from special interests or attempts at manipulation.

All of the terms we have introduced are broad, as each encompasses innumerable perspectives that would deserve more detailed scrutiny. For our purposes here, interest centers on how recursive the aspects we are dealing with have proven to be, and on the frequent swings between well- and ill-founded ideas of medicine and treatment. We intend, then, to reflect on this heterogeneity and the difficulty in mapping where it has gone and where it is going—many ideas and experiments have gone astray or are barely remembered—as we attempt to increase our ability to analyze the problems that stand in the way of an efficient system for safeguarding the right to health.

4 The conceptions of science and of those who establish their coordinates

As Table 4.1 shows, four broad categories of attitudes arise at the intersections of our two dimensions.

Table 4.1 The analytical space

	Binding normative conceptions	*Plural conceptions*
SCIENCE	**1** Scientism Dogmatism Segmentation of the fields of knowledge and hyperspecialization	**4** Validation and hybridization between perspectives (a) within the same discipline (open to exchanges between specializations) (b) among different disciplines
ANTI-SCIENTISM	**2** Negation (in practice) of scientific findings or intuitions in the name of authority: (a) outside the domain of science (b) in the domain of science	**3** Relativism concerning the validity of assumptions or the methods for verifying them Pseudoscience Anti-science populism

4.1 Indisputable conceptions of science

The first cell contains ideas defined as scientific on the basis of binding norms. This set—though internally heterogeneous—is held together by the idea that only certain perspectives are grounded in fact, and all others are invalid. These accepted approaches include, for example, those that embrace scientism, or

> the view that knowledge obtainable by scientific method exhausts all knowledge . . . that whatever is not mentioned in the theories of science [generally thought to mean the physical and experimental sciences] does not exist or has only a subordinate, secondary kind of reality.
>
> (Stevenson & Byerly, 2000, pp. 246–247)

This dogmatic and reductionist attitude denies *a priori* that other standpoints and methods can be contemplated. Attitudes of this kind—based on ideological premises, principles or theories—can be found in many periods of history, not only in moments marked by the growing institutionalization of science and the spread of positivist notions of progress that promised to increase the ability to control reality, anticipate the future and accomplish things that once had been the merest pipe dreams. Interestingly, the idea of one true science by no means prevented tiffs and squabbles among scientists, for instance between those who held, with Comte (1798–1897), that it was necessary to "insist that science is reliable not by virtue of the character of its practitioner, but by virtue of the nature of its practices" (Oreskes, 2019, p. 23). Far from narrowing the field, in fact, attempting to establish what might be a "justified true belief" led to stark contrasts: according to the logical positivists, an observation was true if it could be verified empirically, whereas according to the falsificationists, whether observations are true depends on whether they can be falsified:

> I may have seen one hundred swans, or one thousand, or ten thousand, and found that they have all been white, as have all the swans observed by my scientific colleagues. Therefore, my colleagues and I conclude (seemingly with robust warrant) that all swans are white. Yet, one day I travel to Perth, Australia, where I see a black swan.
>
> (Oreskes, 2019, p. 27)

On the basis of the principle of falsifiability, it is only at this point that we can formulate a statement that meets the criteria of science and say that not all swans are white.

Given our scope here, we can do no more than note that there is more to the story than this, and naturally the two approaches we have mentioned do not reflect the only differences in what constitutes robust proof for science. Epistemological thinking no longer centers on methods alone, but extends to the internal relationships in the community of scientists and to their expectations. For our purposes, suffice it to say that establishing what the foundations of knowledge may be, even in the same scientific community, is far from straightforward. The inability to reach agreement can even be a by-product of scientific advances, for example, when they bring both benefits and unexpected effects. In healthcare, the increase in knowledge that makes it possible to intervene on minute parts of the organism with ever-greater precision has not always helped bring about a more all-encompassing view of the illness and the patient. The consequences of having no common language that enables different competencies to communicate with each other are especially serious in the case of chronic disease or comorbidity.

More generally, we can see that dogmatic visions emerge and re-emerge cyclically, driven by progress in understanding reality and accompanied by the idea that we can sail smoothly toward a hypothetical, unceasing improvement in our living conditions and control over adverse events. It is interesting to note that this is true not only in the boom times, the forward-looking moments but also in occasions of particular uncertainty—catastrophes and pandemics, for instance—when our inability to face the problem's implications and live with the fact that it will not go away seems to fuel our need for firm facts and assurance, not only from those who produce science but also from non-experts, rather than making us more open to looking for ways out of the crisis.

4.2 Indisputable conceptions of authority

In the second cell, we have conceptions that can be labeled as anti-science which—in practice—though running counter to the principles and methods of science, nevertheless claim to lay down the boundaries of what is considered licit and correct in science as well as in other spheres. They also include ideas and conceptions that take dogmatic attitudes based on certain assumptions and principles falling outside the domain of science, as well as others within that domain. Unlike the conceptions in the first cell, here the contrasts do not concern the methods or the legitimacy granted to certain perspectives and denied to others on the basis of specific validation procedures, but the legitimacy of those whom it is believed should decide what is true or false, and what consequently can or cannot be questioned. Here we have the many disputes that have pitted science and theology against each other, and that—not, alas, so very infrequently—resulted in the death of whoever dared oppose the reigning notions. For example, Hellman (2001) tells us of a Scottish lady of rank who had sought relief from the pain of childbirth and was burnt at the stake in 1591 for this attempt to avoid what Holy Writ calls "the primeval curse on woman": the idea that birth must necessarily be associated with the mother's pain. Even when the face-off leaves no room for debating the empirical foundations of the competing positions, the point here is not the content of the disputes but the role of those who hold the power to decide. The beliefs that a particular authority pronounces to be true—regardless of whether or not they are well-founded—cannot be impugned because to do so would mean challenging the role of those who have been given the power to decide what can be considered legitimate. In such circumstances, as Foucault (1985) points out, parrhesia—the capacity to speak *truth* to power and thus intentionally oppose the assumptions regarded as valid and binding in a certain context by calling undisputed dogmas into question—involves taking considerable risks and even—if necessary—putting one's very life on the line.

Accordingly, even where none of the participants in the dispute was actually able to claim a thorough knowledge of whatever underlying physical or physiological processes were involved or their causal mechanisms, one of the positions was often able to assume the status of official truth, while the other was branded as blasphemous or punished for being antithetical to long-established custom and practice. The execution of Giordano Bruno in 1600 is emblematic of the trials carried out by the courts of the Inquisition—over several centuries—which sought to crush heresy by forcefully opposing any idea that could be taken as an alternative to the one hierarchy of the possible, as established by the Church. Hundreds of thousands of trials were held throughout Europe, with countless victims of the religious intolerance that punished anyone who defied recognized authority. While such episodes have undeniably been devastating for the history of mankind over the centuries, for our purposes here it is interesting to look at the more recent past and its instances of opposition to the precepts of science, even within science itself.

These disputes have not been between approaches based on data and evidence, and other conceptions that rely on unprovable or imprecise assumptions. Often, the upper hand has been gained by those who—under the banner of tradition, custom or a particular interpretation of authority—have fought new knowledge provided by scientific insights or new tools for investigating physical and physiological phenomena. Nevertheless, we must not forget that, as Kuhn (1962) pointed out nearly 60 years ago, paradigm change is always been preceded by resistance to accepting new perspectives and ideas and that consequently a certain reluctance to look for solutions outside the established paradigms is inevitably part of research practice (Oreskes, 2019). But let us have a look at some examples of the circumstances that can arise in this cell of our matrix.

In 1628, the physician William Harvey announced that he had discovered how blood circulates, maintaining that the heart was nothing more than a pump that pushes the fluid to all parts of the body. His views were regarded as a shocking attack on the anatomists of the time, who believed, on the basis of ideas that had remained unchanged for centuries, that the movement of the blood was volatile rather than regular, responding to a range of bodily movements, and that the arteries and veins were two independent systems with no communication between them. But Harvey's announcement was not precipitous. His ideas stemmed from a decade and more of research on many animal species, which gave him the solid empirical evidence for proving that the blood circulated between the veins and arteries, though "the optical equipment of his time was not sharp enough to detect the microscopic passages between the arteries and the veins in the extremities" (Hellman, 2001, p. 9). Harvey's story is only one of the many that remind us that new ideas struggle for acceptance, however solid a discovery's foundations may be. A couple of centuries later, the physician Ignaz Philipp Semmelweis succeeded in defeating puerperal fever in 1848, by suggesting that his colleagues simply wash their hands in a solution of chlorinated lime. His ideas were rejected by the Academy of Medicine in Paris, despite the drastic reduction in mortality rates in the maternity wards where his method was applied (Céline, 1952).

These examples, drawn from a much larger pool, invite us to reflect on the fact that significant discoveries—capable of dramatically improving the lives of many people—can go unnoticed if they are not made by the "right" people. As our next story shows, the passage of time has done nothing to change these dynamics.

Thus, closer to our own day, two Australian researchers in the early 1980s discovered that duodenal ulcers, a non-fatal but very painful condition affecting 10% of the world's population, are not caused by poor eating habits or unhealthy lifestyles, as had long been thought, but by a type of bacteria—*Helicobacter pylori*—and could thus be readily diagnosed and cured with a simple and inexpensive course of antibiotics (Heath & Heath, 2007). What makes this discovery—and this story—especially interesting to us here is that, even though the two researchers had presented the scientific community with the evidence and the empirical basis supporting their theory, their findings attracted no interest and were not considered reliable. The two researchers, convinced of their discovery's importance, went to extreme lengths to see that it garnered the attention they felt it deserved: after years of bootless efforts, one of them decided to be his own guinea pig. After an endoscopy to show that his stomach was normal, and as his colleagues watched, he drank a bacterial brew—a suspension of two culture plates—in a scientifically controlled setting. When after a few days he began to show ulcer symptoms, he treated himself with a course of antibiotics and quickly returned to his usual health. Even then, however, the demonstration—and thus the discovery of a cure for ulcers—was not considered credible. Some 15 years were to pass from the time the researchers identified the bacteria responsible for ulcers to the time the impact of their findings was publicly acknowledged: a very long time—with sizable costs for the community and for ulcer sufferers—in the course of which the resources deployed to mitigate ulcer sufferers' symptoms could have been better and more effectively used elsewhere. Fortunately, the researchers' tale had a happy ending, and in 2005, two decades after their discovery, Barry Marshall and Robin Warren were awarded the Nobel Prize in medicine in belated recognition of their work.

4.3 Unbelievable beliefs and concurrent epistemologies

The third cell consists of a constellation of perspectives whose common thread is the idea that there are no absolute truths (or if there are, they are not necessarily produced by experts) and that attempts to limit alternatives can often mask self-interested or manipulative intentions. Pseudoscience—defined as "a pretended or spurious science; a collection of related beliefs about the world mistakenly regarded as being based on scientific method or as having the status that scientific truths now have"[3] —is a label applied, though not without conflict, to approaches each of which claims to embody the only route to truth. Some of these perspectives seem to be unanimously decried by scientists as unfounded; others inspire fierce battles as to whether or not they fall under the heading of science. Here again, the contrast and controversies are long-standing. Sternberg (1897)—whose studies of the causes of malaria and certain forms of pneumonia, and confirmation of the role of the bacilli of tuberculosis and typhoid fever, make him one of the fathers of modern bacteriology—sees the distinction as clear, though he acknowledges that medical science is at once unfinished and an incredibly promising enterprise:

> Thus, astrology, alchemy, phrenology, homeopathy and "Christian Science" have met with acceptance not only by the ignorant, but by many of the so-called educated class. As a matter of fact, a scholastic and classical education does not greatly aid in the differentiation between science and pseudo- science; and at the present day many persons who belong to the "educated class" and even to the learned professions are led astray by claims made upon what appears to them to be a scientific basis. Unless the spirit of scientific scepticism, which demands absolute demonstration before final acceptance, has been cultivated by special training, there is always a liability to be misled by the specious claims of pseudo-scientific pretenders, or of the still more dangerous charlatans who believe in themselves and their pseudo discoveries.
>
> (Sternberg, 1897, p. 202)

What Sternberg grasped over a century ago is that the difficulty of telling the two spheres apart is not just a matter of whether we are experts or not. As he points out:

> [E]ven among those who have had a more or less complete scientific training it often happens that there is a natural tendency to generalize from insufficient data and to jump at conclusions in advance of the experimental evidence which alone could justify them.
>
> (1897, p. 202)

Here again, we could cite many instances of protracted disputes about pseudo-science, some where the label is attached to those who base their conclusions on incomplete evidence; others attempting to take advantage of the ill and their vulnerabilities. We will look at two. The first concerns vivisection and the controversy about the effectiveness of animal experimentation; the second involves some equally controversial cancer treatments.

Medical science has sparred over the use of animals in research since 1865, when Claude Bernard wrote in its favor in a methodological text (Mamone Capria, 2003). Leaving ethical questions aside, from the scientific standpoint vivisection—the practice of testing drugs, treatments and chemical or physical agents on live animals in order to extrapolate the findings to human beings—has been undermined by extensive empirical evidence. As regards toxicity, for example, certain substances have been shown to be: (a) lethal for humans but broadly tolerated by various animal species (like scopolamine, which is harmless to dogs and cats; strychnine, which guinea pigs, chickens and monkeys can take in amounts; and hemlock, which goats, sheep, and various kinds of bird relish or (b) poisonous to some species of animals (dogs, foxes and turkey) but not to people, as in the case of sweet almonds (Mamone Capria, 2003). For those who hold that animal testing is not scientific, problems of generalizability even within the same species and the contradictory results of experiments compel the following conclusions:

> Experiments on animals, because of the differences in reactions across species and the lack of reproducibility even within the same species, lend themselves to being used as pseudo-justification for *any* biomedical hypothesis about man: but they can in no way serve as its rational foundation. It should thus be clear that, if there are reasons to continue animal experimentation, safeguarding *health is not one of them*. Indeed, health is severely jeopardized by the normative accreditation granted to vivisection. We have seen that, as has now been acknowledged officially, *there are no scientific assessments of vivisection's reliability in toxicology and pharmacology which would justify such accreditation.*
>
> (Mamone Capria, 2003, p. 25, emphasis in original)

Though both sides of the vivisection debate claim that their approach is scientific and should be recognized as such, no consensus has ever been reached. In February 2021, Italy's Council of State ruled that testing on rhesus monkeys as part of the *LightUp* project conducted by the Universities of Torino and Parma could be resumed after the moratorium that the *Lega Antivivisezione* (LAV)—an Italian animal rights association recognized by the country's government—had requested in 2020.

The second example—the so-called Hamer method for treating cancer—does not seem to divide the community of scientists, though something of a stir has been caused by pronouncements maintaining that large investments should be channeled into exploring its implications: "We encourage governments and research foundations to give funding in the promising area of holistic cancer treatment a high priority; many patients now want this kind of treatment as it is becoming increasingly popular" (Ventegodt et al., 2005, p. 99). On the website of the Italian Association for Cancer Research, the Hamer method—also known as Germanic New Medicine—and its variant Total Biology are described as practices that are:

> based on a set of theories that have never been submitted to serious scientific testing. The dubious premise is that cancers result from a psychic conflict. In addition to being unfounded, the method's principles deny everything that has been scientifically proven about the functioning of the healthy and diseased organism. . . . The Hamer method eschews the use of pharmaceuticals,

causing patients who follow it to delay treatment until it is too late, turning curable cancers into incurable forms.[4]

Here the question concerns the credibility assigned to oncological approaches that are almost unanimously condemned as anti-scientific by the medical community, although Hamer himself was a physician until he was barred from practicing. Even if new diagnostic abilities have dramatically increased survival rates over the years, cancers continue to be among the public's most feared diseases (Vrinten et al., 2014). Partly because of these fears, illness makes patients extremely vulnerable to messaging that raises hopes in miraculous treatments and equally miraculous cures. Even without attempting to plumb whatever presumable depths of bad faith or profiteering may lie beneath such messaging, its consequences and the uncertainties it often brings to the public discourse are undoubtedly dramatic. How often have we heard of people who died because they suspended treatment in favor of unproven remedies, even in the case of cancers their doctors felt were curable?

In conclusion, then, the duel between science and pseudoscience shows how difficult it is to lay down stable and uncontested boundaries. We must thus proceed with caution in exploring science's assumptions (remember the curse of knowledge?) and the reasons that make it so hard to agree on their credibility, as we will see in a moment when we turn to the approaches in the fourth cell of our matrix.

4.4 Incremental processes

In the fourth and last cell, the conceptions of science are based on the idea that it can only be defined through a necessary and inevitable sequence of trial and error. This theoretical model of science and knowledge is open to thinking about its assumptions and questions them when evidence falsifying their hypotheses comes forth.

The approaches in this cell base their dialog on the most advanced state of knowledge available at a given time and in a given context, aware that this knowledge and the findings stemming from it are provisional. Science is seen as "a process that starts from a problem, tries to solve it and, to do so, formulates conjectures which must then be put to the test through *ad hoc* experiments" (Ferraris, 2017, p. 151). This is a world ideally concentrated on content, where relationships and power are not at the center stage. The quest for middle ground between approaches, including those that are very far apart, seeks integration if it seems promising and consistent with the goal of maximizing patient wellbeing and the more general process of knowledge. Here we find clinical/diagnostic and research approaches that apply self-reflexive methods to their findings and the developments they may lead to, at times through cross-fertilization from other areas. The following examples present attempts to blend dissimilar approaches.

The first example concerns the star-crossed betrothal of evidence-based medicine and narrative medicine. The two perspectives are only apparently opposed, as they have a common need to find the best way of collecting information about the patient's condition and thus improve diagnosis and care. It is interesting to note, moreover, that the gap between the two approaches is more a question of how they are practiced and interpreted by clinicians than of their basic assumptions (Waters & Doyle, 2002). As a group of physicians who support the evidence-based approach emphasize:

> The practice of evidence based medicine means integrating individual clinical expertise with the best available external clinical evidence from systematic research. By individual clinical expertise we mean the proficiency and judgment that individual clinicians acquire through clinical experience and clinical practice. Increased expertise is reflected in many ways, but especially in more effective and efficient diagnosis and in the more thoughtful identification and compassionate use of individual patients' predicaments, rights, and preferences in making clinical decisions about their care.
>
> (Sackett et al., 1996, p. 71)

For its part, narrative medicine has not recognized the need for integration only out of a desire to legitimize this perspective in the eyes of reluctant physicians. There are also more substantive reasons:

> Appreciating the narrative nature of illness experience and the intuitive and subjective aspects of clinical method does not require us to reject the principles of evidence based medicine. Nor does such an approach demand an inversion of the hierarchy of evidence so that personal anecdote carries more weight in decision making than the randomised controlled trial.
>
> (Greenhalgh, 1999, p. 325)

Much can be learned from an approach that can integrate seemingly distant perspectives. For example, it makes it possible to come to grips with the often underestimated phenomenon of clinical disagreement, when physicians dispute each other's diagnoses and treatments: "those of us who practise medicine in a clinical setting, know all too well that clinical judgments are usually a far cry from the objective analysis of a set of eminently measurable 'facts'" (Greenhalgh, 1999, p. 323). Integration can debunk the myth of the objectivity that comes with big numbers, as it shows us what can be accomplished through different vantage points which acknowledge that flights from interpretation in clinical practice are doomed to fail:

> The shadow on the chest radiograph of a 19 year old student returning from an overland trip across India may be objectively identical to that of a 56 year old smoker who has never been out of Sweden. Both may have coughed up blood. But the radiologist who looks at the x ray films "sees" tuberculosis in one and a high probability of cancer in the other.
>
> (Greenhalgh, 1999, p. 325)

Alongside clinical knowledge in the strict sense, approaches such as narrative medicine accentuate—but do not idealize—the co-construction of illness and treatment implicit in the patient–care provider relationship by emphasizing its importance and weight in all phases of illness: determining whether a diagnosis can be reached, for instance, or encouraging better compliance with treatment. Likewise, communication between patients and care providers results in clinical approaches that are better suited to meeting each patient's specific needs. As chronic illnesses increase and disease conditions change, the conception of care that becomes possible enables complex treatment responses to be identified, which puts growing emphasis on knowing about patients' individual and social characteristics and the networks they can rely on for help in facing the stresses of illness.

Our second example concerns treatment protocols that include traditional, but appropriately validated, remedies. In this connection, the WHO published a report in 2010 detailing 28 common ailments that can be treated with traditional herbal remedies that are readily accessible in countries where the most innovative treatments are often out of reach because of their cost. In this case, traditional knowledge joins forces with modern pharmacology's ability to identify the active chemical constituents of each herbal remedy, specifying the dosages, modes of administration and correct use according to the type of ailment and the patients' characteristics. Together, this information can help encourage the widespread use of low-cost medicines that have traditionally been found effective and have also been scientifically validated thanks to the knowledge of each substance and its effects. As the website presenting the report notes:

> It is an attempt to promote the rational, safe and appropriate use of herbal medicines and mainstreaming of traditionally used herbal remedies. This manual can be used by health planners, policy makers, national and district health authorities and others involved in the health sector development and reform. It is also an attempt to increase availability and accessibility to cost-effective treatment of commonly encountered health problems with herbal remedies.
>
> (WHO, 2010).

Though our division of the analytical space into four cells is intended only as an opportunity for reflection, it does show that if anti-scientism continues to be a force opposing science it is not only because of the public's lack of science literacy, as the knowledge deficit theory has long held (Castelfranchi & Pitrelli, 2007; Simis et al., 2016). Even among scientists, as we have seen, refusing to accept methodological assumptions or agree on the importance of certain issues is not unknown, nor are the decisions to reject or embrace new findings or unfamiliar viewpoints on the basis of considerations that have nothing to do with their content or the evidence, such as the characteristics of the researchers involved, the institutions where the discoveries were made, or the need to uphold a certain pecking order in the field.

The four-cell division can also provide a more nuanced picture of certain aspects of the pandemic that have sparked considerable discussion. Recent studies have shown that what we think we know about Covid deniers, conspiracy theorists and anti-vaxxers is in turn the result of stereotypes or unproven theories. This is a central point, and one to which we will return in the conclusions to this chapter. At times, science communication itself seems to see its role as that of a dispenser of knowledge in the shape of a mere list conveying *objective* facts which—sooner or later—must necessarily be recognized as such.

What specific forms do information, error and ignorance take in each of the parts of our analytical space? And what are the features of the communication processes in them? We will address the first question in the following section, while the chapter's conclusions will draw together the many threads we have followed, offering some final considerations about the nexus between communication and health. Discussing what does not attract our attention, what we do not know or do not want to know helps shift our focus to the negatively defined and the seen-but-unnoticed in a way that "reverses the epistemological polarity between figure and ground" (Scott, 2018, p. 4).

5 What we know, what we don't know and how these affect communication

Before attempting to position specific instances of what we do not know in our analytical space and turning to how this affects the forms communication can take, a few words are in order concerning the study of ignorance. Agnotology, as the discipline has been dubbed, has steadily gained recognition over the years (Proctor & Schiebinger, 2008), though not without a certain terminological confusion (Gross, 2007). Abbott reminds us that the study of ignorance and its ramifications has had a number of illustrious forebears—Francesco Petrarca's *De Ignorantia* in 1367, for example—and that starting in the last century sociology and the philosophy of social science (Schneider, 1962) have also directed attention toward it, although "the rarity of these articles suggests a certain sociological ignorance of ignorance" (Abbott, 2010, p. 174). Reflecting on the side of knowledge hiding in the shadows can enrich the history of science and our conceptions of health and illness by providing a complementary vantage point, no longer limited to "the modes of replacing ignorance by knowledge", but open to observing "the formation of a useful kind of ignorance, as distinct from the manifestly dysfunctional kind" (Merton, 1987, pp. 6–7). As we will see, studying ignorance's proliferating meanings can shed light on the risks and opportunities facing the actors who try—not always consciously—to master its effects. The process, provided we can untangle its coordinates, yields a steady stream of surprises, plot twists and unexpected consequences, leading to no preordained outcome: "it's not enough to confess one's ignorance, the point is to specify it" (Merton, 1987, p. 8).

As mentioned earlier, the four cells of our matrix can be taken either as heterogeneous sets of ways of knowing reality or equally varied conceptions of what we do not know. This has specific implications for how health communication is approached and what can legitimately be expected of it.

In the first cell, at the intersection of science and normative conceptions, what we still do not know is polarized. If one of the first ways of framing ignorance is associated with what is considered to be the inevitable march toward greater knowledge and its mirror image, the shrinking boundaries of what we do not know, given the particular view of science taken in this cell, it may well be that the experts themselves unwittingly contribute to producing ignorance. Hyperspecialization, in fact, can mean a failure to see the bigger picture. This problem is not insignificant nor are its implications. In the late 1970s, Leichter used an Indian folktale to illustrate the kind of situation that can result, in this case among scholars of public policy:

> [F]our blind men . . . are led to an elephant. Each is positioned at a different part of the animal: One feels the elephant's leg, another the tail, the third an ear, and the last one the body. As a result of their tactile experiences, each in turn describes what he has felt as a log, a rope, a fan, and a wall.
>
> (1979, p. 8)

Details, details, but no overall understanding: too many trees and not enough forest. An example in medicine is the neglect of gender in clinical trials which, by focusing entirely on male physiology, have assumed that a single part can represent the whole. Despite extensive investigation of the safety and efficacy of drugs, a fundamental and, one would think, obvious point has long been ignored: to establish the correct dosage of a drug, it is not sufficient to consider the relationship between its active ingredients and such characteristics of the individual as weight, age and medical condition. Other often overlooked factors—like the differences in male and female physiologies—can make a major difference in drug uptake, the incidence of adverse drug reactions (ADRs) or reactions to external events (pollution, for instance) and their combination (Holdcroft, 2007; Franconi & Campesi, 2011). Here, ignorance has a cost: knowing about these connections would not only have benefited patients and led in general to a greater knowledge of physiological processes that would have had advantages for everyone, but it also would have made treatments less expensive. While this might seem secondary, it should be borne in mind that (especially where resources are scarce) being able to prevent complications and adverse effects optimizes treatment times and organization, with major repercussions on patients' ability to recover and, obviously, their wellbeing.

Given that the type of knowledge that a dogmatic view of science seeks is highly selective, many opportunities are precluded. This is not always out of "inattentiveness".

The result of selecting what to ignore leads to a contradiction between saying that new knowledge is being sought but at the same time ruling out certain methods in practice, because they are not considered consistent with that particular vision of science and its tools for investigating reality. In this connection, Oreskes speaks of "methodological fetishism", whereby "investigators privileged a particular method and ignored or discounted evidence obtained by other methods, which, if heeded, would have changed their minds" (2019, p. 134). Among the many cases she illustrates, Oreskes tells of scientists' refusal to acknowledge the connection between using the pill and depression, citing the lack of robust epidemiological data, and in particular not recognizing the value—and empirical validity—of women's self-reporting. As she points out: "This doesn't mean that daily experience is superior to statistics" (2019, p. 134), but ignoring its implications, and thus not investigating further, for example, meant that the importance of the link between hormonal contraception and mood disorders was underestimated for decades, to the considerable detriment of many people—and not just women.

In the second cell, at the intersection of anti-scientism and binding conceptions, what perspectives and content are ignored depends on who decides and thus has to do with authority and power. Proctor and Schiebinger (2008) present a number of examples of what is at stake here. When European monarchs and trading companies sent voyagers out in search of fame, fortune and goods a few centuries ago, not all of the knowledge encountered along the way was thought worthy of notice. Much was intentionally suppressed, branded as "superstitions and lies of the devil", as was the case in Diego de Landa's destruction of the Mayan royal libraries on the Yucatan in 1562 (Proctor, 2008, p. 8). Plants such as "cinchona"—quinine—or *Peruvian bark*, used for its anti-malarial properties, or cacao beans, believed to be a specific for stomach upset and consumption, potatoes, rhubarb and many others were part of a flourishing trade in "exotic" products that were all the rage in the European courts of the day. Though the list of natural remedies whose use spread in Europe was long, one that was not included was the "peacock flower", *Poinciana pulcherrima*: "a highly political plant, deployed in the struggle against slavery throughout the eighteenth century by slave women in the West Indies, who used it to abort offspring who otherwise would have been born into bondage" (Schiebinger, 2008, p. 150). Though abortion did not become illegal in Europe until the nineteenth century, knowledge of the peacock flower's use as an abortifacient was rebuffed—an instance of "ignorance as lost realm", or selective choice that Schiebinger attributes to a wide range of circumstances, including the idea that the working class should be numerous, as well as the fact that colonial enterprises were almost exclusively male, and interest thus centered on medicines to protect traders, planters and trading company troops—all groups with few women among them. As many feminist scholars have pointed out, the practices of repression involving women's health, reproduction, body and sexuality based on "knowing that we do not know but not caring to know" (Tuana, 2006, p. 4) have continued down to our own day. The intentional repression of these aspects has profound consequences: "knowledge about what is not known, but considered as unimportant or even dangerous—can lead to non-knowledge" (Gross, 2007, p. 751).

Intentionality, arrogance and the claim that certain matters are irrelevant create needlessly impoverished cultural atmospheres where ignorance is a selective choice (Boaventura de Sousa, 2009), and knowledge that could have proved precious is forever lost.

In the relativism of our third cell, ignorance—in the sense that knowing and agreeing on basic assumptions are regarded as unimportant—is the key factor in arenas that eschew procedures based on consensus. Here as elsewhere, ignorance can take different shapes. It can, for example, be used strategically or self-servingly by those in positions of power: "cultivating ignorance is often more advantageous, both institutionally and personally, than cultivating knowledge" (McGoey, 2012, p. 555). One of the cases that have been most extensively investigated in the literature concerns the use of research data that, over the years, have established the ties between tobacco use and public health risks. Here, we must be careful to separate genuine ignorance from what Galea (2015) calls "manufactured ambiguity", i.e., all the information willfully omitted or artfully falsified in the service of special interests (Norström et al., 2020). The tobacco multinationals relied on their ability to sow confusion by casting doubt on science's findings, clamoring for more proof, more studies, keeping the question of tobacco's hazards for public health open for as long as possible while they continued with unregulated sales of their products. They were thus able to take advantage of a specific form of ignorance, intentionally fomented through well-packaged doubt: "The tobacco industry was rarely innocent in any of these respects, since its goal at many points was to *generate* ignorance—or sometimes false knowledge—concerning tobacco's impact on health" (Proctor, 2008, p. 13).

We can also put a different conception of ignorance in this cell, one which, as we will see, presents significant challenges for communication. The point here, as Oreskes notes, has to do with the fact that for many people the problem is not one of scientific evidence—and so they cannot be convinced on these grounds—but of whether the evidence agrees with the values they hold. It is on this basis that the ideas about health risks are often accepted or rejected:

> The scientific evidence of anthropogenic climate change is clear—as is the evidence that vaccines do not cause autism. . . —but our values lead many of us to resist accepting what the evidence shows.
>
> (Oreskes, 2021, p. 154)

Anti-scientism may not spring from a rejection of science and its methods, but from mistrust of those who produce science, doubts about their integrity and objectivity, the perceived distance from religious or political ideas, or the fear that financial interests may be behind science's choice of subject matter. When such attitudes are ingrained, even communication from experts hoping to increase knowledge and build science literacy may prove fruitless. We will come back to this in the conclusions to the chapter.

The fourth and last cell is that of archetypal Science with a capital S. Here, ignorance is very much a part of the process of coming to know, a boundary that recedes as knowledge advances, continually beckoning us onwards toward new goals. Modernity brings a sort of urgency to this process, where ignorance becomes a void to be filled. From this standpoint, ignorance "can be seen as a *resource*, or at least a spur or challenge or prompt . . . needed to keep the wheels of science turning" (Proctor, 2008, p. 5).

To remind us of what the cognitive enterprise is all about, Merton uses the expression "specified ignorance": "[t]he express recognition of what is not yet known but needs to be known in order to lay the foundation for still more knowledge" (1971, p. 191). Once it has recognized what we do not yet know, science's gaze can turn to new lines of research, breaking down problems into their component parts and identifying the alternatives to be tested.

6 Conclusions: the manifold connections in health communications

The shortcomings of the idea that it is easy to decide what deserves to be communicated in science, and that any difficulties there may be are simply a question of packaging the message appropriately or educating the potential audience, have long been apparent. Dividing the analytical space into four cells has shown, however schematically, how widely varied the situations that can be encountered are. Observing representations of health while bearing the problem of ignorance in mind has helped us narrow our focus among the many factors that make communication between institutions and the public so problematic and concentrate on the lack of clarity, the doubt and uncertainty and the fact that research findings can lead to contradictory or even opposite conclusions. Ignorance is thus inevitable when dealing with processes in constant change. As Galea (2015) argues, we must find ways "to be comfortable in the grays", which can also mean training everyone, experts and non-experts alike, to accept uncertainty as something that cannot be avoided. We must remember—and this is by no means applies only in the field of health—that any innovation (a new molecule, for example, whose potential and effects are still unknown) must be approached through trial and error, with no *a priori* expectations of certainty. We should also remember that expecting uncertainty does not justify inaction and that in many cases a course of action must be chosen without having all the necessary information at hand. Though it might seem contradictory, it is necessary to be absolutely open about uncertainty. As the pandemic demonstrates, thinking that we can put decisions off until we have collected all the evidence or until even the skeptics have been convinced—about the possible benefits of lockdown strategies, for example—can be counterproductive, increasing the number of people exposed to the virus, or of deaths that could have been avoided through faster, albeit uncertain, action. However, we must also recognize—to cite Galea (2015) once again—that acting on the basis of false certitude (or rather, what we believe to be certain but is later found to be wrong) is not without consequences. Being able to test our knowledge against empirical evidence and revise our conclusions is thus especially important. Over and above their inevitable impact on public health, the outcomes of false certitude erode the public's trust in science and reduce the resources available for tackling important problems.

As the conceptions of science and health change, and with them the relationships between the actors straddling the boundaries between what we know and what we do not know or choose to ignore, so change the responsibilities assigned to each actor and the features of the communication among them.

In spheres where hierarchies of methods (cell 1) or roles (cell 2) result in vertical relationships, communication consists essentially of conveying information selected by the experts and serving their goals. In the first cell, communication takes place mostly between communities of experts who share the same orientation or may be intended to delegitimize outsiders. The leadership in dealing with emergencies or specific health conditions claimed by—or granted to—the experts spills over into the realm of communication, and it is thus up to the experts (or so it is felt) to decide what will be communicated, what will be concealed and how and when this will be done. But as we have said, deciding not to communicate or glossing over the reasons behind a decision has consequences, and is tantamount to telling the audience that they are not important, thus fueling their distrust of science.

Communication addressed to non-experts is here largely normative and prescriptive, with no need to establish specific relational modes. In medicine, this may mean that responsibility is assigned entirely to the care providers, while the patients' role is limited to that of compliance, i.e., of following the instructions physicians see fit to give.

In the second cell, communication is even more diluted and centers chiefly on the punishments meted out to whoever opposes dogmas that must not be questioned. Here again, those who hold power are able to decide what is legitimate and what is not. Communication is predominately implicit and in any case top-down, with no way of discussing its content or exchanging views.

In the third cell, communication can be a strategic resource, carefully crafted to win support and stand out among the many proposals, conceptions and approaches that battle for attention in this domain. Communication in the fourth cell is the mainstay of the ties and exchanges between experts and approaches that are needed to pursue the goal of increasing knowledge in the community of scientists and facilitating its dissemination among the general public.

Though we have gone into each dimension in considerable detail, there are still many aspects of science and health communication that merit further exploration. Here we will do no more than mention them, as a suggestion for future research.

Much has changed since 1985, when the Bodmer Report (Bodmer, 1985) ushered in a new era in the Public Understanding of Science (PUC). As Castelfranchi and Pitrelli (2007) note, the report regards communication as primarily a question of translating complex concepts which, in order to fulfill the educational function of science and knowledge, must be made comprehensible to an essentially ignorant public. This outlook seems to run counter to much of what we have discussed in the foregoing pages: even in the late 1800s, as we saw in Section 4.3, Sternberg (1897) and others had already called the idea of one-way scientific communication into question, holding that the division between experts who know and the public that knows nothing does not reflect the facts on the ground. And yet, the so-called knowledge deficit model, with its linear (and unrealistic) view of how knowledge is transmitted continued to raise its head (Simis et al., 2016) over and over again in the subsequent decades. Surveys carried out in the United States, Europe and the rest of the world over the years have shown "that the number of people who can be considered 'science literate' continues to be low and has not varied with time" (Castelfranchi & Pitrelli, 2007, p. 68). Though the effort and the resources channeled into communication have increased, the results still fail to come up to expectations.

Once again, we find ourselves wondering why certain ideas that have been shown to be wrong are so difficult to change and seem indeed to reproduce almost through inertia.

The idea of experts versus non-experts tells only part of the story. The growing number of actors involved has reframed the field of health communication, making it ever more complicated and at times confused. As Briggs and Hallin emphasize, biomedicalization, through "the expansion of the social and cultural influence of biomedicine", has brought additional complications:

> biomedicalization is a complex process, entailing internal changes in biomedical fields as, for example, research science and pharmaceutical industries become more powerful relative to individual clinicians. It also involves increased interpenetration between medicine and other social fields as medicine has become entangled with the market and the state, and more central to forms of governance.
>
> (Briggs & Hallin, 2016, p. 16)

The result has been a greater "heterogeneity of production, distribution, and access to biomedical knowledges" (Clarke et al., 2003, p. 177). Along with this process, an expanding number of media outlets have, here as elsewhere, brought a proliferation of sources carrying information about science and the interests involved (Ahmed & Bates, 2013). At the confluence of biomedicalization and mediatization,[5] we see once again that the communicative relationship is more like a tangle of wires of many different shapes and sizes than a cable running straight between two poles.

But the complications do not end here. Many scholars have found that the public is farther than ever from being a uniform, uninformed mass devoid of health literacy: views of science are as varied as the population itself. An Italian survey of the participants in a nationwide protest against mandatory pediatric vaccines in 2017, for example, noted that "the problem is not so much one of mistrust in science per se" as it is of "the skepticism about how scientific activity is organized, especially as regards setting priorities and allocating resources, given the widespread perception that market considerations and financial interests carry considerable weight in such matters" (Lello, 2020, pp. 489–490). Out of a sample of around 500 participants in the protests, the survey found that the percentage of people with tertiary and upper secondary levels of education was markedly higher than in the population as a whole (44% and 44% as against 14% and 30% of the total Italian population in 2017). According to the researchers, this indicates "something quite different from the anti-scientific attitude" and which involves a belief in non-conventional and alternative practices or—on the part of a second group of interviewees who habitually rely on conventional medicine but combine it with alternative practices chiefly for preventive purposes—opposition to the fact that vaccinations are mandatory rather than to vaccination as such (Lello, 2020, p. 492). Many people seem to espouse concurrent epistemologies that combine a criticism of certain aspects of biomedicine with the desire "to actively exercise their personal right/duty of control" over their own conduct and their own choices. Top-down communication—as envisaged by the knowledge deficit model—shows itself to be increasingly unable to connect with a variegated and constantly changing public. Though attempts are underway to pass from the PUS model to broader-based approaches to dialog between lay people and experts like Public Engagement with Science (PES), we can no longer simply assume that communication will be a straightforward, linear process. Explaining the relationship between information and misinformation (Wang et al., 2019) in ways that go beyond thinking only in terms of rationality and irrationality calls for an untiring capacity for reflection and analysis.

All of us, experts included, have a vision very like that of the four blind men who can only feel a very limited part of the elephant. The challenge is to put the whole picture together, knowing that, as Oreskes' message about trusting science reminds us, making good decisions means integrating many kinds of information (2021). This is a never-ending enterprise. And it is inevitably social and collective, requiring efforts from all of us, each with our own bit of the elephant.

Notes

1 Preamble to the Constitution of the World Health Organization as adopted by the International Health Conference, New York, June 19–22, 1946; signed on July 22, 1946, by the representatives of 61 States (Official Records of the World Health Organization, no. 2, p. 100) and entered into force on April 7, 1948.
2 As we saw in Chapter 1, the successes logged in public health are only partly due to the contribution of medicine in the strict sense. To a larger extent, they have stemmed from changing living conditions and the more general improvement in hygiene and diet that have gradually spread among the population. Nevertheless, science and its advances continue to receive the greatest credit.
3 Oxford English Dictionary, www.oed.com/
4 www.airc.it/cancro/informazioni-tumori/corretta-informazione/nuova-medicina-germanica-metodo-hamer
5 A term coined by Briggs and Hallin, *biomediatization* is a process that is not just about the production of articles, broadcasts, websites, and tweets, that is, things that are contained with the sphere of "the media": basic notions of health, disease, citizenship, immigration, ethno-racial categories, and of "the state" are also getting constructed in the process. (2016, p. 13).

References

Abbott, A. (2010). Varieties of Ignorance. *The American Sociologist, 41*, 174–189. https://doi.org/10.1007/s12108-010-9094-x.

Ahmed, R., & Bates, B. (Eds.). (2013). *Health Communication and Mass Media*. London: Routledge. https://doi.org/10.4324/9781315586335.

Armaroli, P., Battagello, J., Battisti, F., Giubilato, P., Mantellini, P., Sassoli de Bianchi, P., Senore, C., Ventura, L., Zappa, M., & Zorzi, M. (2020). *Rapporto sui ritardi accumulati alla fine di maggio 2020 dai programmi di screening Italiani e sulla velocità della ripartenza*, August. www.osservatorionazionalescreening.it/content/rapporto-ripartenza-screening-maggio-2020.

Austin, J. L. (1962). *How to Do Things with Words*. Oxford: Oxford University Press.

Badash, I., Kleinman, N. P., Barr, S., Jang, J., Rahman, S., & Wu, B. W. (2017). Redefining Health: The Evolution of Health Ideas from Antiquity to the Era of Value-Based Care. *Cureus, 9*(2), e1018. https://doi.org/10.7759/cureus.1018.

Bambra, C., Riordan, R., Ford, J., & Matthews, F. (2020). The COVID-19 Pandemic and Health Inequalities. *Journal of Epidemiology and Community Health, 74*(11), 964–968. https://doi.org/10.1136/jech-2020-214401.

Beyerstein, B. L. (1996). *Distinguishing Science from Pseudoscience*. Department of Psychology- Simon Fraser University. www.dcscience.net/beyerstein_science_vs_pseudoscience.pdf.

Bianchi, C. (2021). *Hate Speech. Il lato oscuro del linguaggio*. Roma-Bari: Editori Laterza.

Blumer, H. (1971). Social Problems as Collective Behavior. *Social Problems, 18*, 5.

Boaventura de Sousa, S. (2009). A Non-Occidentalist West? Learned Ignorance and Ecology of Knowledge. *Theory, Culture & Society, 26*(7–8), 103–125. https://doi.org/10.1177/0263276409348079.

Bodmer, W. (Ed.). (1985). *The Public Understanding of Science*. London: Royal Society.

Bosco, N. (2012). *Non si discute. Forme e strategie dei discorsi pubblici*. Torino: Rosenberg & Sellier.

Bourdieu, P. (1982). *Ce que parler veut dire. L'économie des échanges linguistiques*. Paris: Librairie Arthème Fayard. English translation by Gino Raymond, & Matthew Adamson (1991), *Language and Symbolic Power*. Cambridge, MA: Harvard University Press.

Briggs, C., & Hallin, D. (2016). *Making Health Public*. London: Routledge. https://doi.org/10.4324/9781315658049.

Butler, J. (1997). *Excitable Speech. A Politics of Performative*. London: Routledge.

Canguilhem, G. (1966). *Le normal et le pathologique*. Paris: Presses Universitaires de France. English translation by C. R. Fawcett, & R. S. Cohen (1989), *The Normal and the Pathological*. Zone Books.

Castelfranchi, Y., & Pitrelli, N. (2007). *Come si comunica la scienza?* Bari: Editori Laterza.

Céline, L. F. (1952). *Semmelweis (1818–1865)*. Paris: Édition Gallimard.

Ciofi, R. (2015). Verso una nuova definizione del concetto di salute—Oltre la definizione dell'OMS. *Pol.it- Psychiatry Online Italia*. www.psychiatryonline.it/node/5605.

Clapp, J. D., Lange, J. E., Russell, C., Shillington, A., & Voas, R. B. (2003). A Failed Norms Social Marketing Campaign. *Journal of Studies on Alcohol, 64*(3), 409–414. https://doi.org/10.15288/jsa.2003.64.409.

Clarke, A., Shim, J., Mamo, L., Fosket, J., & Fishman, J. (2003). Biomedicalization: Technoscientific Transformations of Health, Illness, and U.S. Biomedicine. *American Sociological Review, 68*(2), 161–194. www.jstor.org/stable/1519765.

Cochrane, A. L. (1972). *Effectiveness and Efficiency: Random Reflections on Health Services*. London: Nuffield Provincial Hospitals Trust.

Colombo, E., & Rebughini, P. (Eds.). (2003). *La medicina che cambia. Le terapie non convenzionali in Italia*. Bologna: il Mulino.

Conrad, P., & Barker, K. K. (2010). The Social Construction of Illness: Key Insights and Policy Implications. *Journal of Health and Social Behavior*, *51*(1_suppl), S67–S79. https://doi.org/10.1177/0022146510383495.

D'Agostini, F. (2010). *Verità avvelenata. Buoni e cattivi argomenti nel dibattito pubblico*. Torino: Bollati Boringhieri.

Engel, G. L. (1977). The Need for a New Medical Model: A Challenge for Biomedicine. *Science, New Series*, *196*(4286), 129–136. https://intranet.newriver.edu/images/stories/library/stennett_psychology_articles/Need%20for%20a%20New%20Medical%20Model%20-%20A%20Challenge%20for%20Biomedicine.pdf.

Farre, A., & Rapley, T. (2017). The New Old (and Old New) Medical Model: Four Decades Navigating the Biomedical and Psychosocial Understandings of Health and Illness. *Healthcare (Basel, Switzerland)*, *5*(4), 88. https://doi.org/10.3390/healthcare5040088.

Ferraris, M. (2017). *Postverità e altri enigmi*. Bologna: il Mulino.

Foucault, M. (1963). *Naissance de la Clinique. Une archeology du regard medical*. Paris: Presses Universitaires de France. English translation by Alan Sheridan (1973), *The Birth of the Clinic: An Archaeology of Medical Perception*. London: Tavistock Publications.

Foucault, M. (1971). *L'Ordre du discours*. Paris: Éditions Gallimard. English translation by Ian McLeod (1981), The Order of Discourse. In Young, R. (Ed.), *Untying the Text: A Post-Structuralist Reader*. Boston and London: Routledge & Kegan Paul.

Foucault, M. (1985). *Discourse and Truth. The Problematization of Parrhesia*. Evanston, IL: Northwestern University Press.

Foucault, M. (1999). *Les Anormaux. Cours au collège de France. 1974–1975*. Paris: Seuil/Gallimard. English translation by Graham Burchell (2003), *Abnormal. Lectures at the Collège de France, 1974–1975*. London and New York: Verso.

Franconi, F., & Campesi, I. (2011). Farmacologia di genere. *Bollettino SIFO Società Italiana Farmacia Ospedaliera*, *57*(3), 157–174. https://doi.org/10.1704/932.10219.

Frank, A. F. (2013). *The Wounded Storyteller. Body, Illness, and Ethics*, Second Edition. Chicago and London: The University of Chicago Press.

Freidson, E. (1970). *Profession of Medicine: A Study of the Sociology of Applied Knowledge*. New York: Harper & Row.

Galea, S. (2015). *On Ignorance and Public Health, Dean's Note*. Boston University School of Public Health, 20 September. www.bu.edu/sph/2015/09/20/on-ignorance-and-public-health/.

Glaser, B. G., & Strauss, A. L. (1965). *Awareness of Dying*. New York: Aldine Transaction.

Goffman, E. (1961). *Asylums. Essays on the Social Situation of Mental Patients and Other Inmates*. New York: Anchor Books, Doubleday & Company, Inc.

Golding, P., & Middleton, S. (1982). *Images of Welfare. Press and Public Attitudes to Poverty*. Oxford: Basil Blackwell.

Greenhalgh, T. (1999). Narrative Based Medicine: Narrative Based Medicine in an Evidence Based World. *BMJ (Clinical research ed.)*, *318*(7179), 323–325. https://doi.org/10.1136/bmj.318.7179.323.

Gross, M. (2007). The Unknown in Process: Dynamic Connections of Ignorance, Non-Knowledge and Related Concepts. *Current Sociology*, *55*(5), 742–759. https://doi.org/10.1177/0011392107079928.

Gusfield, J. R. (1989). Constructing the Ownership of Social Problems: Fun and Profit in the Welfare State. *Social Problems*, *36*(5), 431–441. https://doi-org.eres.qnl.qa/10.2307/3096810.

Heath, C. (2003). Loud and Clear. Crafting Messages that Stick—What Nonprofits Can Learn from Urban Legends. *Stanford Social Innovation Review*. https://ssir.org/articles/entry/loud_and_clear#.

Heath, C., & Heath, D. (2007). *Made to Stick. Why Some Ideas Survive and Others Die*. New York: Random House.

Hellman, H. (2001). *Great Feuds in Medicine. Ten of the Liveliest Disputes Ever*. New York: John Wiley and Sons. https://doi.org/10.1136/jech-2020-214401.

Hirshman, A. (1991). *The Rhetoric of Reaction. Perversity, Futility, Jeopardy*. Cambridge, MA: The Belknap Press of Harvard University Press.

Holdcroft, A. (2007). Gender Bias in Research: How Does It Affect Evidence Based Medicine? *Journal of the Royal Society of Medicine*, 1–6. www.ncbi.nlm.nih.gov/pmc/articles/PMC1761670/.

Huber, M., Knottnerus, J. A., Green, L., van der Horst, H., Jadad, A. R., Kromhout, D. et al. (2011). How Should We Define Health? *British Medical Journal*, *343*. https://doi.org/10.1136/bmj.d4163.

Hyman, H., & Sheatsley, P. (1947). Some Reasons Why Information Campaigns Fail. *The Public Opinion Quarterly*, *11*(3), 412–423. Retrieved 7 February 2021, from www.jstor.org/stable/2745237.

Jensen, N., Kelly, A. H., & Avendano, M. (2021). The COVID-19 Pandemic Underscores the Need for an Equity-Focused Global Health Agenda. *Humanities and Social Sciences Communications*, *8*, 1. https://doi.org/10.1057/s41599-020-00700-x.

Kleinman, A., Eisenberg, L., & Good, B. (1978). Culture, Illness, and Care: Clinical Lessons from Anthropologic and Cross-Cultural Research. *Annals of Internal Medicine*, *88*(2), 251–258. https://doi.org/10.7326/0003-4819-88-2-251.

Kuhn, T. S. (1962). *The Structure of Scientific Revolutions*. Chicago: The University of Chicago Press.

Leichter, H. M. (1979). *A Comparative Approach to Policy Analysis: Health Care Policy in Four Nations*. Cambridge: Cambridge University Press.

Lello, E. (2020). Populismo anti-scientifico o nodi irrisolti della biomedicina? Prospettive a confronto intorno al movimento free vax. *Rassegna Italiana di Sociologia*, *3*, 479–508. https://doi.org/10.1423/98558.

Lidler, E. L. (1979). Definitions of Health and Illness and Medical Sociology. *Social Science & Medicine. Medical Psychology & Medical Sociology*, *13*(6), 723–731. https://doi.org/10.1016/0271-7123(79)90118-4.

Lupton, D. (1993). Risk as Moral Danger: The Social and Political Functions of Risk Discourse in Public Health. *International Journal of Health Services*, *23*(3), 425–435. https://doi.org/10.2190%2F16AY-E2GC-DFLD-51X2.

Mamone Capria, M. (2003). Pseudoscienza nella scienza biomedica contemporanea: il caso della vivisezione. *Biologi Italiani*, *6*, 10–27. http://docplayer.it/12451244-Pseudoscienza-nella-scienza-biomedica-contemporanea-il-caso-della-vivisezione.html.

Martini, A., & Falletti, V. (2005). La valutazione dei risultati delle campagne di comunicazione sociale: questioni di metodo e studi di casi. In Cucco, E., Pagani, R., & Paquali, M. (Eds.), *Primo Rapporto sulla Comunicazione sociale in Italia*. Roma: Rai-Eri, 179–220.

McGoey, L. (2012). The Logic of Strategic Ignorance. *British Journal of Sociology*, *63*(3), 553–576. https://doi.org/10.1111/j.1468-4446.2012.01424.x.

Merton, R. K. (1971). The Precarious Foundations of Detachment in Sociology. In Tiryakian, E. A. (Ed.), *The Phenomenon of Sociology*. New York: Appleton-Century-Crofts, 188–199.

Merton, R. K. (1987). Three Fragments from a Sociologist's Notebooks: Establishing the Phenomenon, Specified Ignorance, and Strategic Research Materials. *Annual Review of Sociology*, *13*(1), 1–29. https://doi.org/10.1146/annurev.so.13.080187.000245.

Neresini, F. (2001). Salute, malattia e medicina: lo sguardo sociologico. In Bucchi, M., & Neresini, F. (Eds.), *Sociologia della salute*. Roma: Carocci.

Newton, L. (1990). *Overconfidence in the Communication of Intent: Heard and Unheard Melodies*. Unpublished doctoral dissertation. Stanford, CA: Stanford University.

Norström, J., Thunström, L., Van't Veld, K., Shogren, J., & Ehmke, M. (2020). Strategic Ignorance of Health Risk: Its Causes and Policy Consequences. *Behavioural Public Policy*, 1–32. http://doi.org/10.1017/bpp.2019.52.

Oreskes, N. (2019). *Why Trust Science?* New York: Princeton University Press.

Parsons, T. (1951). *The Social System*. London: Routledge & Kegan Paul.

Peters, M. A. (2020). Anti-Scientism, Technoscience and Philosophy of Technology: Wittgenstein and Lyotard. *Educational Philosophy and Theory*, *52*(12), 1225–1232. https://doi.org/10.1080/00131857.2019.1654371.

Proctor, R. N. (2008). Agnotology: A Missing Term to Describe the Cultural Production of Ignorance (and Its Study). In Proctor, R. N., & Schiebinger, L. (Eds.), *Agnotology. The Making & Unmaking of Ignorance*. Stanford, CA: Stanford University Press, 1–33.

Proctor, R. N., & Schiebinger, L. (Eds.). (2008). *Agnotology. The Making & Unmaking of Ignorance*. Stanford, CA: Stanford University Press.

Rosenbaum, L. (2020). The Untold Toll—The Pandemic's Effects on Patients Without Covid-19. *The New England Journal of Medicine*, *82*, 2368–2371. https://doi.org/10.1056/NEJMms2009984.

Rosenstock, I. M. (1974). Historical Origins of the Health Belief Model. *Health Education Monograph*, *2*(4), 328–335. https://doi.org/10.1177/109019817400200403.

Sackett, D. L., Rosenberg, W. M. C., Gray, J. A. M., Haynes, R. B., & Richardson, W. S. (1996). Evidence Based Medicine: What It Is and What It Isn't. *British Medical Journal*, *312*, 71. https://doi.org/10.1136/bmj.312.7023.71.

Saracci, R. (1997). The World Health Organisation Needs to Reconsider Its Definition of Health. *BMJ (Clinical Research ed.)*, *314*(7091), 1409–1410. https://doi.org/10.1136/bmj.314.7091.1409.

Scamuzzi, S., & Tipaldo, G. (Eds.). (2015). *Apriti scienza. Il presente e il futuro della comunicazione della scienza in Italia tra vincoli e nuove sfide*. Bologna: il Mulino.

Schiebinger, L. (2008). West Indian Abortifacients and the Making of Ignorance. In Proctor, R. N., & Schiebinger, L. (Eds.), *Agnotology. The Making & Unmaking of Ignorance*. Stanford, CA: Stanford University Press, 149–162.

Schneider, L. (1962). The Role of the Category of Ignorance in Sociological Theory: An Exploratory Statement. *American Sociological Review*, *27*(4), 492–508. www.jstor.org/stable/2090030.

Scott, S. (2018). A Sociology of Nothing: Understanding the Unmarked. *Sociology*, *52*(1), 3–19. https://doi.org/10.1177/0038038517690681.

Seale, C. (2003). Health and Media: An Overview. *Sociology of Health & Illness*, *25*, 513–531. https://doi.org/10.1111/1467-9566.t01-1-00356.

Simis, M. J., Madden, H., Cacciatore, M. A., & Yeo, S. K. (2016). The Lure of Rationality: Why Does the Deficit Model Persist in Science Communication? *Public Understanding of Science (Bristol, England)*, *25*(4), 400–414. https://doi.org/10.1177/0963662516629749.

Smith, R., & Rennie, D. (2014). Evidence-Based Medicine—An Oral History. *JAMA*, *311*(4), 365–367. https://doi.org/10.1001/jama.2013.286182.

Stacy, A. W., Bentler, P. M., & Flay, B. R. (1994). Attitudes and Health Behavior in Diverse Populations: Drunk Driving, Alcohol Use, Binge Eating, Marijuana Use, and Cigarette Use. *Health Psychology*, *13*(1), 73–85. https://doi.org/10.1037//0278-6133.13.1.73.

Sternberg, G. M. (1897). Science and Pseudo-Science in Medicine. *Science*, *5*(110), 199–206. https://science.sciencemag.org/content/5/110/199.

Stevenson, L., & Byerly, H. (2000). *The Many Faces of Science: An Introduction to Scientists, Values and Society*. Boulder, CO: Westview Press.

Teixeira da Silva, J. A. (2020). Stigmatization, Discrimination, Racism, Injustice, and Inequalities in the COVID-19 Era. *International Journal of Health Policy and Management*, *9*(11), 484–485. https://doi.org/10.34172/ijhpm.2020.87.

Tuana, N. (2006). The Speculum of Ignorance: The Women's Health Movement and Epistemologies of Ignorance. *Hypatia*, *21*(3), 1–19. www.jstor.org/stable/3810948.

van Dijk, T. A. (2006). Discourse and Manipulation. *Discourse & Society*, *17*(3), 359–383. https://doi.org/10.1177/0957926506060250.

van Doorn, J., Verhoef, P. C., & Bijmolt, T. H. A. (2007). The Importance of Non-Linear Relationships Between Attitude and Behaviour in Policy Research. *Journal of Consumer Policy*, *30*, 75–90. https://doi.org/10.1007/s10603-007-9028-3.

Ventegodt, S., Andersen, N. J., & Merrick, J. (2005). Rationality and Irrationality in Ryke Geerd Hamer's System for Holistic Treatment of Metastatic Cancer. *The Scientific World Journal*, *5*, 93–102. https://doi.org/10.1100/tsw.2005.16.

Vrinten, C., McGregor, L. M., Heinrich, M., von Wagner, C., Waller, J., Wardle, J., & Black, B. B. (2014). What Do People Fear About Cancer? A Systematic Review and Meta-Synthesis. *The Lancet*, *384*, 12. https://doi.org/10.1016/S0140-6736(14)62138-3.

Wang, Y., McKee, M., Torbica, A., & Stuckler, D. (2019). Systematic Literature Review on the Spread of Health-Related Misinformation on Social Media. *Social Science & Medicine*, *240*, 112552. https://doi.org/10.1016/j.socscimed.2019.112552.

Waters, E., & Doyle, J. (2002). Evidence-Based Public Health Practice: Improving the Quality and Quantity of the Evidence. *Journal of Public Health*, *24*(3), 227–229. https://doi.org/10.1093/pubmed/24.3.227.

Will, C. M. (2020). The Problem and the Productivity of Ignorance: Public Health Campaigns on Antibiotic Stewardship. *The Sociological Review*, *68*(1), 55–76. https://doi.org/10.1177/0038026119887330.

World Health Organization. Regional Office for South-East Asia. (2010). *Traditional Herbal Remedies for Primary Health Care*. WHO Regional Office for South-East Asia. https://apps.who.int/iris/handle/10665/206024.

Conclusion
Knowledge about the past and discourses about the future

The situation in India—where people are dying by the thousands and there were 380 casualties in the capital on April 26, 2021 alone—seems to show how little we've learned slightly over a year since the pandemic began. The BBC News website shows images of the makeshift funeral pyres set up in Delhi's parks after the city's crematoriums were overwhelmed and families have had to wait hours and hours before cremating their dead.

In all their force and violence, these images "regarding the pain of others" (Sontag, 2003) make us think about how it is that the information and representations we are exposed to are able to reach us, build up in us and become part of our own experience, and about how we might be able to turn them to use in refocusing attention on improving public health. Like many of the things we have talked about in this book, these problems are not new, though they often continue to seem as if they were. In the last century, and especially around the time of the Holocaust, many scholars have delved into the relationship between knowledge and action, into what we do—individually and collectively—with the knowledge theoretically available to us, into how communication can influence our awareness and into how and why we decide to accept or deny its implications (Bloch, 1969; Cohen, 2001). While accumulated experience has undeniably changed, this has not brought any increase in the collective capacity for memory that could help us deal with the things that seem problematic to us, or even any greater awareness of our inability to remember. Exposure to suffering and health inequalities, how we sidestep them or meet them head on, and the models and solutions we devise for handling their implications all involve a relationship between information, knowledge and choices that is much less linear than we think. We continually forget that we forget.

Understanding what really makes us able to react to what is or seems to us to be socially unexpected is not easy, not even after events that have once again shaken the very foundations of many of our certainties. But there is still room for a few considerations that can clarify the approach taken in this book and suggest future routes for exploring the mechanisms currently at work in healthcare as a result of our societies' growing interdependencies and the role that the social sciences can play in helping us understand them.

1 More about the links between information, knowledge, communication and choices

We know many more things about the pandemic than we did a year ago, for example, about the virus' characteristics and how to curb its spread, or about how the disease evolves and the strategies to adopt in treating patients at various stages of illness. As Oreskes (2019) points out, we have good, solid reasons for trusting science, which, in this particular circumstance, has pulled off an unprecedented and immensely important feat in developing effective vaccines at a speed that would have been unthinkable just a few years back. Alongside these conquests, and despite our greater knowledge, old problems persist, and we are no better able to take effective evidence-based action, for instance, by formulating global strategies to block the virus' spread so that variants are less likely to evolve. The knowledge built up in this past year has not prevented the population in many parts of the world from laboring, even now, under enormous difficulties aggravated by the pandemic, with no access to hospitals and treatment, no basic equipment and materials and not enough oxygen to prevent patients from suffocating to death or at least ensure that they can end their days without undue and avoidable suffering. We have the vaccines, but at the same time, we still cannot make them effectively available to everyone, everywhere. We speak of health as a public good, but we do not know how to regulate the immense private profits it yields. Big Pharma has received billions in public funding and guaranteed pre-orders for Covid vaccines, but according to the data collected in 2021 by the NGOs Oxfam and Emergency, both members of the People's Vaccine Alliance:

> Ahead of shareholder meetings for the giant pharmaceutical corporations, the People's Vaccine Alliance calculates that Pfizer, Johnson & Johnson and AstraZeneca have paid out $26 billion in dividends and stock buybacks to their shareholders in the past 12 months. This would be enough to pay to vaccinate at least 1.3 billion people, the equivalent of the population of Africa.[1]

Knowledge and ignorance, strategic messaging and unwitting or unintentional disclosure are opposites we have come across frequently in these pages, and which have mingled in varied and often unexpected ways throughout the history of science, public health and our more or less adequate efforts in these areas. The fact that such striking contradictions are still largely unresolved, and our persistent inability to see the bigger picture brings us back to a point we have mentioned several times: the gap between the information we have, and the possibility that this information can circulate, become an asset for all and enable us to formulate strategies, make informed decisions and explain the rationale behind them.

To address at least some of healthcare's complexities and ambivalences—which the pandemic has made all the more acute—we have attempted to provide an "exploded" view of the many mechanisms at work in the field, and, in so doing, take the lid off the black box of the things we tend to take for granted (Zerubavel,

2018). As we have seen, wicked problems and dilemmas abound. For one thing, the fact that there are so many different actors involved—all with different interests and objectives and powers—and so many shifts in the balance between public and private, as well as in the role of the multinationals and of politics, has meant that the types of organization employed by healthcare systems, the resources available to them and how equally or unequally these resources are distributed are likewise varied. But the most disconcerting aspect, at least in the present writer's opinion, is not that the attention paid to health inequalities and the differences between healthcare systems is so incredibly uneven. Rather, it is the fact that whatever form a particular system takes, there is always a pronounced tendency to take that form as right and normal, forgetting or ignoring that other possibilities exist. Even when change presents itself as an option spurred perhaps by extreme events like the pandemic, it can at times fall back on habitual patterns out of a form of half-conscious inertia. Retracing some of the passages in the history of science and medicine has been what we might call an exercise in rememory (De Leonardis, 2001), enabling us to present a much less linear view of the ideas and practices that have accompanied the world of health and its inhabitants. We have thus found ourselves face to face with changes whose meaning is often neither clear nor what we would have expected. In addition to the changing conceptions of health and illness, the varying weight assigned to acute and chronic conditions and how treatment is organized accordingly, we have looked at the many different ways of using information to support choices and the array of criteria applied in collecting data in ranking healthcare systems or deciding how to allocate resources. We have also seen that there is a gap between what we think we know and what we really know, between what is voiced publicly and what is never said out loud. As is often the case, close scrutiny of any object, any phenomenon raises more questions than answers. And the road we have taken in this volume has brought us up against many unexpected twists and turns—unexpected even for the writer—that have demonstrated how difficult understanding the mechanisms at work here continues to be. For example, the quality of a system may be assessed without specifying how judgments are arrived at, and when judgments are favorable it may be that scores are used as if they were absolutely synonymous with the quality they are intended to measure. Or it may be that there is a yawning gulf between what is publicly communicated and what actually happens in practice. Painfully emblematic of these disconnects are the situations when decisions must be made about who will and will not receive scarce resources or the violation of the most fundamental human rights (to life, to health and to non-discrimination) of the many elderly people who were essentially abandoned to die in care homes, in Italy as elsewhere (Amnesty International, 2020): all of which was publicly denied or repressed in the public consciousness.

What vantage points can help us make progress in not only preserving but also making radical changes in a public good which—like health—is now more important than ever?

In these few final pages, we will reflect on the areas where our certainties were most shaken, and on what is needed in order to shore them up. But first, we will try to turn the usual questions on their heads: What did we *not* learn? What did we *not* see? What did we avert our eyes from, and what mechanisms—apart from the many different special interests involved—can help us understand why we did so? How did we picture science and its goals? What tools do we have to understand the changed view of care providers, who, in a few short months, went from being heroes to sharing the blame for what went wrong?

2 Why we are never ready

As we have seen, it is not easy to agree in principle about what a quality health-care system should be like, even though many of the suggestions for how to leave the pandemic behind us seem to accept some of the same priorities (fairness, equality or personalized treatment, for instance) and embrace the same forms of communication. Recent studies of communication strategies in situations of high uncertainty have emphasized that it is counterproductive to ignore this uncer-tainty and its implications. Quite the opposite is necessary, in fact. Uncertainty should be disclosed, and we must be open about our limitations: "Part of telling the whole story is talking about what we don't know" (Blastland et al., 2020). The fact that experts' competence may be acknowledged does not appear to be enough to ensure they are regarded as trustworthy unless there is also clarity about their motivations, their honesty and their doubts and conflicts. And they must also be able to admit their mistakes, as some have striven to do. Smith et al. (2020), for example, concluded a recent editorial dealing with the need to acknowledge uncertainty with a statement about what they had not understood, what they had underestimated and where they had been wrong about Covid-19 in the early stages of the pandemic. They underscored the crucial role that admitting the fallibility of one's viewpoint has in building public trust and determining who deserves it: "When deciding whom to listen to in the covid-19 era, we should respect those who respect uncertainty, and listen in particular to those who acknowledge con-flicting evidence on even their most strongly held views" (Smith et al., 2020).

The most common way of tackling the health emergency, however, has not been that of accepting uncertainty and trying to get a handle on it. At least in the public discourse, attention has mostly centered on strategies for getting ahead of uncertainty so as not to be caught unprepared, as if that meant that we were deal-ing with a succession of purely technical aspects that only needed to be communi-cated in the right way. As we have seen throughout these pages, however, nowhere in the world was foresight and forecasting sufficient to produce the concrete poli-cies, organizational systems and communications needed to face the continual emergencies in public health, though there were a few promising attempts. While it is true that putting abstract principles into actual practice is objectively difficult, it is nevertheless inevitable that the expectations in this area are very high, and the unresolved tension between preparedness and uncertainty merits further thought. These are aspects that call for our attention and open onto new lines of research suggested by the pandemic and the challenges of understanding its mechanisms and social determinants. In these concluding remarks, we will return to three key points—the ambiguity of the concepts involved in healthcare, interdisciplinarity and the need for networked approaches—and to the role that the social sciences can play in understanding their scope.

2.1 Concepts and their layered meanings

Experts, policy makers and the public now seem to agree on the need for an alternative model of healthcare. This call for change is by no means new (Engel, 1977), and what "new" means differs widely from place to place, given the many and varied types of organization and policies in the sphere of health. What kind of change are we talking about? Saying that there is a need is not the same as saying where we should be going, and deciding on the direction and all its implications calls for long hard thought. But though no one seems to deny the need for change; agreeing on the models to be followed and the choices that will make it possible to move in whatever direction the various actors opt for is no simple matter. Sennet (2018) points out that any human construction requires constant upkeep and often repair, both because of wear and tear and because changing conditions may make it necessary to rethink and re-plan what has been done if it is not (or is no longer) able to meet our needs. Though Sennet is concerned with cities, his reflections also apply to changes in any institutional setting. What are the structures, relationships, processes and priorities that we imagine could help improve how healthcare operates and is managed? What changes do we think should be made in how healthcare professionals are trained and work? Establishing who we consider part of *us* and what defines the reasons for change cannot be linked to any single prospect, and clarifying the concepts we use is thus an essential first step, whatever route we intend to take. Let's look a few examples.

Repairing something, Sennet tells us, can take at least three forms, each entailing different operations: the first is restoration, or returning the object in question to its previous condition. Fixing healthcare could mean returning to the pre-pandemic situation, for example, by restoring hospitals to some hypothetical equilibrium they supposedly enjoyed before all this happened, closing the Covid wards and going back to the activities they had performed in treating patients with other ailments. In our case, this is a route that no one seems particularly keen on taking, given that the pandemic laid bare many critical organizational and management problems that had largely avoided notice before.

The second form is remediation, or in other words returning to the earlier situation but using some innovation that has become available in the meantime. In the sphere of healthcare, the innumerable improvements that could be introduced include new systems for booking appointments using the technological infrastructures developed during the period of lockdown, forms of telemedicine and, obviously, many others. With this second set of changes, the situation could be better than it was in some respects, but there would be no substantial differences in its fundamental framework.

The third route—reconfiguration—involves far more sweeping changes in form and structure. Not only are these changes more basic but they are also opened-ended, as they can evolve in many different ways depending on the situation and its constraints, the specific actors involved, their commitment and the balance of power between them, the level of vigilance that civil society can or will exercise, legacy skills, available resources, etc. And it is in this third form of repair, where uncertainty about the directions that could or should be taken reigns, that change cannot depend only on technical abilities. It also calls for a collective reflection—and redefinition, if necessary—on the meaning of action, a tight focus on the objectives to be pursued and a capacity on the part of governments and the international bodies (such as the World Health Organization) to mediate between the needs and interests of the actors involved—Big Pharma, health professionals and caregivers of all kinds, patients' associations, etc.—as well accurate, up-to-date information for measuring the distance between the starting conditions and what we decide to do. Sennet's point concerns the connection between the ethical dimension of change and the careful use of the words we employ: words, he says, are shells of meaning. And we can never assume that there is any single, shared meaning.

Obviously, however, it is not only the ideas that can be associated with change that call for attention and caution. There is much talk about preparedness, a concept we discussed in Chapter 3 and whose exact coordinates are not easy to map out (WHO, 2021). Being prepared, or rather, knowing what to expect, is not simply a question of being able to assemble information (however indispensable that may be) nor does it arise automatically out of an ability to model different options for future action. Indeed, decisions about the future reveal the political nature of how we choose to implement the idea of preparedness, for instance, by opting for risk-taking strategies as opposed to risk-avoidance (Pellizzoni, 2020). These are processes that do not call only for attention to the technical aspects but also bring politics into play and hinge on the ability to visualize the alternatives and determine which course of action will make them practicable. Communication itself and the narratives constructed about what the future may hold contribute to shaping the horizon of possibilities and making it in some degree acceptable and inevitable.

Even the concept of equality, which is frequently said to be one of the goals of rethinking the public health system, is not necessarily self-evident. Different—and not always consistent—ideas of what equality means are rooted in theoretical and practical approaches that can produce very dissimilar sets of circumstances. If, for example, we take equality to mean equality of opportunity, then we must try to ensure that everyone starts off on the same footing, "with an equal likelihood of reaching a given opportunity". Quite a different perspective is opened up if we aim for equality of conditions, "where everyone has the same chance to access a set of basic goods" (Granaglia, 2020, p. 29). In the case of vaccine distribution, equality of opportunity could be achieved by drawing lots to determine who is entitled to the jab, while if our goal is to see that everyone has the same chances of staying healthy—or in other words establish equality of conditions—then it would be necessary to vaccinate the higher-risk categories of the public first.

Similar attention should be given to inequalities and their distribution, identifying the role played by the fundamental institutions of social organization (Gallino, 2000), the weight of the mechanisms of exclusion that the market society can bring to bear and distinguishing them from the forms of "unequal inclusion" produced in society (Burawoy, 2015).

It should be clear at this point just how influential the words we use and the meanings we associate with them are in producing very different courses of action and policy choices. Our ideas of change, of the future and of the goals that merit pursuing exemplify concepts that we use frequently without realizing that they are not self-evident or mean the same thing to everyone. This brings us to our next point and to the need to find new ways of linking knowledge and divergent viewpoints in each of the many spheres involved in safeguarding the collective health.

2.2 The importance of the connection between knowledge and skill

In his exploration of the ethics of the city, Sennet notes that the first attempts to deal with public health when migration swelled Europe's cities in the eighteenth century were not spearheaded by medical professionals. Indeed, doctors as well as the public attempted to combat such emergencies as the great cholera outbreaks with practices that were "rooted deeply in ignorance" (Sennet, 2018, p. 22), with little knowledge of how diseases spread. It was the civil engineers and urbanists who took on the task of improving the quality of city life through technical experimentation: they thus tested new materials and found ways to improve the population's living conditions and sanitation, for example, by using smooth, machined stone paving to make the streets easier to clean. Sennet lists many of the inventions and innovations of those years that made cities healthier places and demonstrated the benefits of taking a more panoramic view of public health, and considering the specific settings. Ideas about the organic causes of the spread of disease were still often based on old wives' tales, like the belief that covering the mouth with a white handkerchief could protect against illness, not because of the covering, but because of the powers of the color white. By contrast, the new urbanists started from the assumption that providing the right infrastructure would encourage people to change their behavior. Thus, for example, when *pissoirs* were installed in Paris in 1834, and "urine could be channelled below ground" (Sennet, 2018, p. 23), the general advance in sanitation resulted in greater public awareness, and city dwellers gradually developed a new sense of shame about relieving themselves in full view. The idea that behavior regarded as conducive to improving individual and collective living conditions could be incentivized has many echoes in what have come to be known as nudge strategies—where a gentle nudge is intended to sway conduct in a direction that is considered more appropriate without seeking to mandate or require such behavior, but simply encouraging it by making certain courses of action easier or desirable (Thaler & Sustein, 2008). This approach has been highly successful over the years and has been equally good at sparking discussion about how controlling the institutions' relationship with the public should be. According to advocates of the nudge, this is a relationship that calls for a sort of libertarian paternalism: a combination of two apparently contradictory concepts, given that those who take a paternalistic attitude usually consider themselves—or are considered by others—as authoritative and in a position to lay down the law. These considerations encourage us to think, not so much about the pros and cons of a particular decision-making process, but about the need to devote time and resources to finding how the different components of society can be engaged in questions of public interest. Different points of view encourage wider reflection, bringing a greater capacity to anticipate effects and consequences, intentional or otherwise, and thus be able to choose and, once again, gain insights into the nature of the changes we would like to see.

Aside from drawing attention to the echoes of past thinking that can be found in new approaches, these examples from bygone times remind us that combining skills that are apparently far apart and not directly connected with health can help in unpacking knotty public problems, as it brings new outlooks and points of view. Over the past year and more, the pandemic has made us more aware of the need to enlist a wider range of skills than those offered by the natural, medical and health sciences, as in the case of the Medical Humanities, where the relationship between health and society is addressed from the many perspectives offered by multiple disciplines. But more must be done. And once again, this is not a new idea. As early as the 1950s, C. Wright Mills pointed out that stating and solving significant problems requires a selection of materials, conceptions and methods from more than one discipline (1959, p. 142). In more recent years, the sociology of innovation has taken this to heart (Ramella, 2013), demonstrating the potentially generative character of integration—or even conflict—between disciplines and perspectives and the importance of precisely those circumstances where uncertainty holds us in its thrall:

> Where the organizational environment is turbulent and there is uncertainty about what might constitute a resource under changed conditions, contending frameworks of value can themselves be a valuable organizational resource. . . . Not the property of an individual personality but, instead, the function of an organizational form, entrepreneurship is the ability to keep multiple principles of evaluation in play and to benefit from that productive friction.
>
> (Stark, 2009, p. 18)

These are points that also apply in public health, where uncertainty need not necessarily result in stasis, but can spur new strategies. Today (or perhaps always), the very idea of health needs to be re-thought and, to gird ourselves for the cultural as well as structural and distributive challenges we face, a plurality of viewpoints can prove enormously useful:

> Epidemics are not solely a function of pathogens; they are also a function of how society is structured, how political power is wielded in the name of public

health, how quantitative data is collected, how diseases are categorised and modelled, and how histories of disease are narrated. Each of these activities has its own history. As historians of science and medicine have long pointed out, even the most basic methodologies that underpin scientific research—observation, trust in numbers, the use of models, even the experimental method itself—have a history. They should not be taken as a given, but understood as processes, or even strategies, that were negotiated, argued for and against, and developed within particular historical contexts and explanatory schemes.

(Charters & McKay, 2020, p. 225)

2.3 *The obstacles to consensus-based solutions*

Whatever each of us may have thought about the public health decisions made during the pandemic and the way they were communicated, the approach taken in this volume should have demonstrated that continual interaction and exchanges between the actors involved at various levels can result in well-grounded positions that can then be put to the test and can produce new ideas by focusing on risks and opportunities. Though dialog is widely seen as desirable, the operations that permit it are difficult to put into practice, and not everyone is convinced that they are worth the effort. As we have seen, science—and, obviously, all the other areas involved in public health—is by no means monolithic, and its internal dialog is a continual juggling of divergent viewpoints and ideas. The importance of starting from "a portrait of science as a communal activity of experts, who use diverse methods to gather empirical evidence, and critically vet claims deriving from it" (Oreskes, 2019, p. 246) is thus called into question even within a community which has shown interest in exploring its implications. The idea that the main thrust of scientific endeavor is not to produce certainty about its findings but to develop processes subject to constant validation and reconsideration by a broad set of actors often yields to the widespread thirst for reassurance.

On the other hand, it is important to note that an increasing number of battle lines are being drawn around public policies, and retracing how this has affected the current pandemic and the many past emergencies is instructive in casting light on the risks of approaches that rely overmuch on one-size-fits-all methods and assume that science can dominate uncertainty. In this connection, an international team of scholars from a number of disciplines (statistics, mathematical modeling, epistemology, history, sociology, epidemiology) recently published a manifesto in the pages of *Nature*, with an appeal not to be led astray by the seduction of numbers but to accept uncertainty, taking a humble attitude and acknowledging ignorance and the importance of transparency in order to ensure that models are used responsibly, both by those who produce them and by those to whom they are addressed:

> Modellers must not be permitted to project more certainty than their models deserve; and politicians must not be allowed to offload accountability to models of their choosing. . . . Mathematical models are a great way to explore questions. They are also a dangerous way to assert answers. Asking

models for certainty or consensus is more a sign of the difficulties in making controversial decisions than it is a solution, and can invite ritualistic use of quantification.

(Saltelli et al., 2020)

If science—and the resulting achievements in public health—is to be truly the outcome of a communal process, all components of society must be actively engaged. This entails complex processes, and how they will end—as we saw from the deliberative experiments discussed in Chapter 3—is never predictable. Patient involvement in resource allocation decisions, for example, is a mantra on many lips, but is hardly a process that can be conjured into existence simply by being invoked, even with the fervent support of the health institutions themselves. The importance assigned to involvement can be seen—not just from the surrounding discourses—but from the resources actually earmarked for achieving it:

> A maxim of contemporary moral philosophy is that "ought" implies "can". It is contradictory for the UK Government to insist that GPs improve their professional practice with patients in specific ways without finding the resources for these improvements to be practically possible. To do otherwise is to engage in empty moral abstraction, in this case about patient participation and involvement in professional decision-making.
>
> (Jones et al., 2004, p. 100)

What, then, does adopting a multidisciplinary approach entail in healthcare? First of all, it means remembering that the relationship between science and society is never neutral; on the contrary, we must "consider the sum total of the intersecting scientific and political dimensions". Factors that are apparently far removed from each other show a tight web of interconnections, and we must be able to trace all of its radiations and ramifications:

> The credibility of producing a drug or a vaccine is not just an internal question circulating among a closed community of scientists, but has a direct impact on the credibility of the pharmaceutical companies listed on the stock market, just as the credibility of a country's public health system is directly linked to the scores assigned to it by the rating agencies.
>
> (Chesta, 2020)

A wide range of analytical abilities is needed to understand the workings of this web of interconnections and grasp the full extent of the global mechanisms and tensions that can have an impact on the ability to meet the public's healthcare needs (Dentico & Missoni, 2021). As these brief concluding remarks have sought to show, the questions circulating in the health arena must be considered in the light of the social and economic conditions that establish their coordinates, linking them to the macro social dimensions (such as the effects of globalization on governance and economic aspects) and their repercussions on all the facets of healthcare, right down to the relationship between providers and patients. We have also seen that how problems are framed affects their visibility and whether or not appropriate resources can be found for communicating the thinking behind them and the implicit assumptions, values, interests and beliefs that influence the choices of the actors involved, which often remain in the shadows. Problem-setting is thus central, and must necessarily come before any attempt at problem-solving, even though it takes time and resources and does not lead to immediate answers. And it is here that sociology and the social sciences in general can make a difference.

The social sciences' potential role

As Duncan Watts—a physicist turned sociologist—reminds us, sociology tends to be looked down upon as a science because it deals with things that seem familiar to us simply because they are part of our own experience:

> If a physicist explains something to you about superconductivity, you may or may not find it interesting but you are not going to dismiss the conclusions as obvious—or as obviously wrong. When the topic is human or social behaviour, however, the feeling that we already understand what is being explained often elicits precisely these reactions.
>
> (Watts, 2011, p. 32)

In reality, the social sciences are concerned with complex phenomena that, by contrast with the no less complex subject-matter of the so-called hard sciences, cannot be studied in isolation: "Unlike in physics, therefore, essentially every problem of interest to social scientists requires them to consider events, agents and forces across multiple scales simultaneously" (Watts, 2011, p. 32). The role of the social sciences in the debate on public health, and more generally on the problems affecting society, is not limited to trotting out to sociological concepts, but presupposes an analytical approach that, starting from such concepts, can shed light on what undergirds the different meanings they produce and probe the latter's implications. This is important when it is necessary to formulate a concrete set of public policies for addressing a particular challenge, not just by redistributing goods and resources but by exploring how these resources can be put to good use in solving the problems at hand.

Though deciding what action should be taken is not up to the social sciences, they can nevertheless be expected to reframe problems, draw on the past thinking about these problems and provide an understanding of the mechanisms that make it difficult to view them from a shared perspective. According to a recent study of the persistence of unfounded beliefs, scientists in the STEM fields (science, technology, engineering, and math) who have also been trained in the social sciences seem less inclined to harbor simplified views or adhere to obsolete models (like the deficit model we discussed in Chapter 4) about the lack of connection between science and society than those who do not have such training (Simis et al., 2016).

The social sciences—often accused of over-problematizing with no real capacity to provide immediate workable answers—can have a role (though not the only role) in improving our ability to understand reality. For example, they shed light on the dramatic inadequacies of collective responses, furnish the theoretical and methodological tools for rewinding the film, as it were, and reviewing how many times we have done the same things and said the same words in the past. They enable us to retrace—using increasingly sophisticated data collection and analysis techniques—trends in inequalities and their exponential growth around the world, as well as to reconstruct the meaning of the concepts we use, the actions we take unthinkingly, and those we take deliberately. The theories of public choice developed in recent decades, studies of the state and institutions, and of the changes wrought in capitalism and globalization, the focus on the dynamics of innovation, network analysis, the reconstruction of public discourses and social representations, political science's studies of power and its interconnection, history's ability to spur reflection about what strikes us as new even if it is not, the opportunities that anthropology and the sociology of culture provide for investigating the plurality of conceptions held by the public and the mechanisms whereby they are naturalized, and explorations of the socially constructed nature of the world are only a few of the tools we now have for observing and analyzing the reality that surrounds us. They encourage us not to take priorities for granted, to observe how and by whom they are defined and re-defined and how they can continue to exist out of inertia. This wide repertoire of practices and interconnections between disciplines and their areas of knowledge is the foundation we need in order to start afresh in developing an ability to analyze the uncertainty that, together with the pandemic we are struggling to control, seems almost suffocating us.

Note

1 Retrieved from: www.oxfam.org/en/press-releases/pharmaceutical-giants-shell-out-billions-shareholders-world-confronts-vaccine

References

Amnesty International. (2020). *UK: Older People in Care Homes Abandoned to Die Amid Government Failures During COVID-19 Pandemic.* www.amnesty.org/en/latest/news/2020/10/uk-older-people-in-care-homes-abandoned-to-die-amid-government-failures-during-covid-19-pandemic/.

Blastland, M., Freeman, A. L., van der Linden, S., Marteau, T. M., & Spiegelhalter, D. (2020). Five Rules for Evidence Communication. *Nature, 587,* 362–364. https://doi.org/10.1038/d41586-020-03189-1.

Bloch, E. (1969). *Spuren.* Frankfurt am Main: Suhrkamp Verlag. English translation by Anthony A. Nassar (2006), *Traces.* Stanford: Stanford University Press.

Burawoy, M. (2015). Facing an Unequal World. *Current Sociology, 63*(1), 5–34. https://doi.org/10.1177/0011392114564091.

Charters, E., & McKay, R. A. (2020). The History of Science and Medicine in the Context of COVID-19. *Centaurus*, *62*, 223–233. https://doi.org/10.1111/1600-0498.12311.

Chesta, R. M. (2020). Neoliberismo, tecnoscienza e democrazia nell'era Covid. *Sbilanciamoci Info-org*. https://sbilanciamoci.info/neoliberismo-tecnoscienza-e-democrazia-al-tempo-del-covid/.

Cohen, S. (2001). *States of Denial. Knowing About Atrocities and Suffering*. Cambridge: Polity Press.

De Leonardis, O. (2001). *Le istituzioni. Come e perché parlarne*. Roma: Carocci.

Dentico, N., & Missoni, E. (2021). *Geopolitica della salute. Covid-19, OMS e la sfida pandemica*. Soveria Mannelli: Rubbettino Editore.

Engel, G. L. (1977). The Need for a New Medical Model: A Challenge for Biomedicine. *Science, New Series*, *196*(4286), 129–136. https://intranet.newriver.edu/images/stories/library/stennett_psychology_articles/Need%20for%20a%20New%20Medical%20Model%20-%20A%20Challenge%20for%20Biomedicine.pdf.

Gallino, L. (2000). *Globalizzazione e diseguaglianze*. Roma-Bari: Editori Laterza.

Granaglia, E. (2020). What Idea of Equality for the Welfare State? Defense of the "Old" Idea of Equality of Conditions, Politiche Sociali. *Social Policies*, *1*, 19–38. https://doi.org/10.7389/97333.

Jones, I. R., Berney, L., Kelly, M., Doyal, L., Griffiths, C., Feder, G., Hillier, S., Rowlands, G., & Curtis, S. (2004). Is Patient Involvement Possible When Decisions Involve Scarce Resources? A Qualitative Study of Decision-Making in Primary Care. *Social Science & Medicine (1982)*, *59*(1), 93–102. https://doi.org/10.1016/j.socscimed.2003.10.007.

Oreskes, N. (2019). *Why Trust Science?* New York: Princeton University Press.

Pellizzoni, L. (2020). The Time of Emergency. On the Governmental Logic of Preparedness. *AIS- Sociologia Italiana*, *16*, 39–54.

Ramella, F. (2013). *Sociologia dell'innovazione economica*. Bologna: il Mulino.

Saltelli, A., Bammer, G., Bruno, I., Charters, E., Di Fiore, M., Didier, E., . . . Vineis, P. (2020). Five Ways to Ensure that Models Serve Society: A Manifesto. *Nature*, *582*, 482–484. https://doi.org/10.1038/d41586-020-01812-9.

Sennett, R. (2018). *Building and Dwelling: Ethics for the City*. London: Penguin Books.

Simis, M. J., Madden, H., Cacciatore, M. A., & Yeo, S. K. (2016). The Lure of Rationality: Why Does the Deficit Model Persist in Science Communication? *Public Understanding of Science*, *25*(4), 400–414. https://doi.org/10.1177/0963662516629749.

Smith, G. D., Blastland, M., & Munafà, M. (2020). Covid-19's Known Unknowns. *British Medical Journal*, *371*, m3979. https://doi.org/10.1136/bmj.m3979.

Sontag, S. (2003). *Regarding the Pain of Others*. New York: Farrar, Straus and Giroux.

Stark, D. (2009). *The Sense of Dissonance: Accounts of Worth in Economic Life*. Princeton and Oxford: Princeton University Press.

Stevenson, L., & Byerly, H. (2000). *The Many Faces of Science: An Introduction to Scientists, Values and Society*. Boulder, CO: Westview Press.

Thaler, R. H., & Sustein, C. R. (2008). *Nudge. Improving Decisions About Health, Wealth and Happiness*. London: Yale University Press.

Watts, D. (2011). Why Everything That Seems Obvious isn't. *Physics World*, *24*(10), 30–34.

WHO. (2021). *COVID-19 Strategic Preparedness and Response Plan*. www.who.int/publications/i/item/WHO-WHE-2021.02.

Wright Mills, C. (1959). *The Sociological Imagination*. Oxford: Oxford University Press.

Zerubavel, E. (2018). *Taken for Granted. The Remarkable Power of the Unremarkable*. Princeton and Oxford: Princeton University Press.

Index

For Product Safety Concerns and Information please contact our EU
representative GPSR@taylorandfrancis.com
Taylor & Francis Verlag GmbH, Kaufingerstraße 24, 80331 München, Germany

www.ingramcontent.com/pod-product-compliance
Lightning Source LLC
Chambersburg PA
CBHW060314220326
41598CB00027B/4328

9 781032 157092